SAVING AMERICA

Saving America

Solutions for A Nation in Crisis

Adel N. Shenouda M.D., F.A.C.P.
with
Frank Sanello

Foreword by the Honorable John Duran,
Mayor of West Hollywood, Calif.

iUniverse, Inc.
New York Lincoln Shanghai

Saving America
Solutions for A Nation in Crisis

iUniverse books may be ordered through booksellers or by contacting:

iUniverse
2021 Pine Lake Road, Suite 100
Lincoln, NE 68512
www.iuniverse.com
1-800-Authors (1-800-288-4677)

ISBN: 978-0-595-48013-5 (pbk)
ISBN: 978-0-595-71511-4 (cloth)
ISBN: 978-0-595-60115-8 (ebk)

Printed in the United States of America

For my grandchildren Laila and Madeline and the grandchildren of all Americans with the hope that they may live in a great country for centuries to come.

—A.S.

For my dear sister and brother-in-law, Evelin and John Knorr.

—F.S.

"Each man must for himself alone decide what is right and what is wrong, which course is patriotic and which is not."

—Mark Twain

Contents

ACKNOWLEDGMENTS

Many thanks to my parents, my wife Brenda, my children Samer, Monica, Christina and Lisa, my grandchildren Laila and Madeline as well as Dr. Sergio Acchiardo, Dr. Phillip Burns, Dr. Don Franklin, Gen Di Napoli, Dr. Dan Fisher, Dr. Claude Galphin, Nikki Hadson, Dr. Fred Hatch, Dr. James Gibb Johnson, Dr. Keith Johnson, Dr. Roger Jones, Sara King, Bertha Miller, Dr. Frank Miller, The Penn Group LLC, Dr. Charles Richardson, David Sadlow, Nancy Smith, Betty Solomon and Dr. Ralph Stafford.

Special thanks to my agent, for believing in my work and David Bird for his invaluable assistance in editing it.

—Adel N. Shenouda, M.D., F.A.C.P.

Many thanks to Daniel Abraham, Kyle Baker, Edith Barcay, A. Scott Berg, Ellen Bersch, Professor Joseph Boone, Dr. Daniel Bowers, Robert Buckley, Charles Casillo, Jim Chud, Louis Chunovic, Dr. Gary Cohan, Dr. Jeffrey L. Conklin, Michael Dardenelle, Ghalib Dhalla, Michael Dorr, Anita Edson, Mike Emmerich, Cyrus Godfrey, Lawrence C. Goldstein, Mary and Art Goodale, André Guimond, Dr. Stephen Graham, Mike Hamilburg, Dr. Scott Hitt, Frederick Hjelm, Brad Kane, Evelin and John Knorr, Pamela Lansden, Robert Lent, Michael Levine, Will Litchfield, Rod Lurie, Christina Madej, Paul Manchester, David Marlow, Kevin Moreton, Jim Murphy, James Robert Parish, Dr. Joshua Penn, Dr. Dale Prokupek, Sia Prospero, Lee Ray, Linda and Phil Reinle, Ray Richmond, Doris Romeo, Marjorie Rothstein, Guy Shalem, Dr. Adel Shenouda, Professor Benjamin

Sifuentes-Jauregui, Dorie Simmonds, Victor Stone, Professor Leon Tho-mas, Christopher Villa Woods, and Jeff Yarbrough.

—Frank Sanello

FOREWORD

Hope For a Nation in Crisis

Reading *Saving America's* discussion in Chapter Four of the madness in Iraq, I found myself recalling a sad event from my past, although the authors' ingenious solutions for leaving Iraq alleviated some of my sadness. Two years ago, when I was a West Hollywood City Councilman, I introduced a resolution that made the city the first in Southern California to go on record opposing the war, long before the situation became so bleak that now even conservative Republican politicians, as Chapter Four says, are— "like rats deserting a sinking presidency"—fearful of their reelection chances in 2008, have defected from President Bush's stubborn refusal to compromise on the war and in the process have defected from the leader of their party himself.

I remember when the City Council of West Hollywood passed the resolution in 2005. The toll of American men and women whose lives had been wasted on an unnecessary conflict had climbed to 2,000, and at the time I thought, "What a terrible benchmark!" Now, fatalities as of June 9, 2007, surpass the 3,500 mark with almost 26,000 more wounded according to iCasualties.org—unthinkable statistics two years ago.

Sadly, as *Saving America* points out, we won't be leaving Iraq until at least the president leaves office—and I fear a long time after that. Bush should have listened to his father who was wise enough not to take Baghdad during the Persian Gulf War in 1991, because, while the elder Bush realized that we could win the war, he also knew that we could not win the peace.

Now, we find ourselves stuck in a lose-lose situation with no exit plan, although Chapter Four suggests a brilliant way to withdraw all American troops ASAP. But until the book's solutions are implemented, if ever, we will continue to waste billions of dollars on mayhem and murder that could have been better expended on homegrown issues like providing affordable health insurance, improving public transportation, restoring our crumbling infrastructure, reducing crime, repairing our broken educational system—all the actions that would have benefited Americans instead of making us the most reviled nation in the world. Billions wasted, thousands of lives lost or ruined, our standing abroad demonized and eviscerated, the country made more, not less, vulnerable to terrorist attacks at home, and all the other effects of the war in Iraq have made it the first tragedy of the 21st Century.

Although it will be a pyrrhic victory, there is a silver lining in the black cloud that Iraq has become. As Chapter One explains, disenchantment with the war will indirectly end Congressional gridlock as voters fed up with the war vote obdurate hawks in the Republican ranks out of office and replace them with enough Democrats to stop filibusters in the Senate and override presidential vetoes.

By the time of the 2008 election, the war will still be on the front burner and hopefully opposition to it will galvanize voters to, as they say in baseball, "throw da bums out."

The introduction of the filibuster process, before it became obstructive of the public will, was prompted by good intentions. The framers of our Constitution purposely intended the Senate to be a deliberative, slow-moving body and set a high hurdle for political change to take place. Our 18th Century Founding Fathers were gentlemen farmers and wealthy merchants who feared mob rule and its demands for for instant legislative gratification. Filibusters served their purpose in slowing anarchic political momentum and allowing issues to be studied and debated at a pace that allowed reflection before action. No bread and circuses, just the slow evolution of our body of law.

Now filibusters do not slow the actions of government; they make it come to a standstill on important legislation for immigration reform, troop withdrawal from Iraq and embryonic stem cell research among many other important issues stalled in both houses of the Federal legislative branch.

At the moment, only the president and his Republican base, including the subset of this group called the ultra right, still do not recognize the folly of the Commander in Chief's adventurism. Fortunately, the ultra right wing's influence is diminishing as evidenced by the Democratic sweep of the 2006 mid-term elections and polls showing that Americans by a large majority believe Democrats will do a better job solving the nation's problems.

Historically, the ultra right in American politics goes through cycles, and currently we are on the downside of a cycle that began in 1980, when Jerry Falwell and his Moral Majority started coalescing the obsessions of the far right into a powerful special interests group by using religious members of the right to push their political agenda.

One sign of the decline of the right was the Teri Schiavo tragedy, described in Chapter Five, where for political rather than compassionate reasons, legislators and the president set aside serious government business to meddle in the private affairs of a grieving family. As the Schiavo case played out, the American people recognized the poisonous impact and influence religious fundamentalists have on policy makers.

The religious far right will use any issue, no matter of how little concern it is to mainstream Americans, to strengthen their political position. In California, they tried in 1978 to pass Proposition Six, the Briggs Initiative, a ballot referendum that would have purged public schools of gay and lesbian teachers, but Californians decided this was a monstrous intrusion into private life and rejected the initiative decisively—but only after Mr. Conservative himself, Ronald Reagan, went on the record opposing it.

Now, fundamentalists are using AIDS and the non-issue of gay marriage to enhance their influence and distract voters from issues that polls show Americans genuinely care about. Whomever they're bullying at the moment, their venom wears thin after a while, and they go on to their next victims, who these days seem to be illegal aliens as conservatives try to pass immigration laws that are unfair and cruel, not to mention unworkable. The far right relies on fear—fear of blacks, gays, immigrants—to build and expand their base. They move from target to target, seeking out society's most vulnerable.

The only way to combat this fear-based strategy is with the facts. For example: opponents of immigration reform should realize that immigrants contribute to the American economy and provide the rich fabric of our national diversity. Keeping facts like that in front of the American people dispels fear. On the issue of marriage equality, despite predictions of the fall of Western Civilization as we know it by the religious right, in places where gay men and lesbians have been given the right to marry, instead of the predicted chaos, we have seen a return to civil order even though marriage equality at one time had been controversial in those countries where it has been legalized.

From Massachusetts to Canada, from Spain to Amsterdam—wherever marriage equality has been established despite the objections of religious fundamentalists, democracies continue to hum along without interruption as the sense of fundamental *fairness* calms the political contortions of the right wing.

The left must participate in diminishing the power of these theocratic demagogues. We have to stop "preaching to the choir," i.e., we need to talk not just to each other—we're already convinced, but we also have to work with the people in the center who hold the balance of power. We will never reach the right with reason or logic because they have isolated themselves in their fear-based world.

Chapter Four tackles an even more intractable problem, the Israeli-Palestinian conflict, but *Saving America's* tough-love approach to the 60-year standoff offers hope. I have my own prescription for peace in the Middle East, but sadly it will take generations before we ever see tranquility in that sanguine part of the world.

The solution revolves around the city of Jerusalem. In order to resolve this hydra-headed issue, the world politic is going to have to accept the proposition that Jerusalem is an *international* city—it doesn't belong to the Jews, Muslims or Christians, but to the entire world. We must set up Jerusalem as a world city that belongs in the global community under that classification.

Both sides need to compromise. Israel must return some of the real estate expropriated from the Palestinians in 1948, 1967 and 1972. In this peace-for-land exchange, Palestinians have to agree to the right of Israel to exist. And instead of the president's unilateralist approach to the civil war in Israel, the U.S. cannot go it alone.

We will never succeed without the cooperation of relatively friendly nations like Egypt and Saudi Arabia and even pariah nations like Syria and Iran. There is an applicable Arab aphorism: Keep your friends close, but your enemies closer. That justifies a hold-your-nose-while-you-shake-hands approach with sponsors of state terrorism like Syria and Iran.

As for the rest of the mess in the Middle East, the solution will be a generational one as it will be for Israel and the Palestinians. The U.S. has a lot of repair work to do in that region, and unfortunately the Bush administration has set us back a generation by its solipsistic belief that we can impose Western-style democratic processes on people with no historical or cultural institutions in place to support a free democratic system in lands that have known only repressive, authoritarian rule for more than a millennium and a half.

We need to treat our Arab and Muslim allies with the same respect we treat our allies in Europe and accept the fact that the system of government in Middle East nations will of necessity be different from ours. Tolerance is the operative word here.

We will never see the crime reduction Chapter Seven proposes until the failed concept of indeterminate sentencing is taken off the books because it imposes maximum and minimum sentencing limits which tie the hands of judges who need to take into account mitigating factors like poverty and mental illness before they hand down their sentences.

As a long-time criminal attorney myself, I have seen how indeterminate sentencing shackles jurists and how it fails to promote the rehabilitative elements of the criminal justice system. Judges are forced to treat criminals like numbers and statistical averages rather than as human beings. Indeterminate sentencing handles the punishment part of justice effectively but contributes nothing to the rehabilitation process.

Judges must be allowed to shake off their handcuffs and be granted greater latitude in sentencing. Remove indeterminate sentencing and you return to the sound notion that the judge's legal reasoning should determine, on humanitarian grounds, what sentence length to impose on a case-by-case basis—the way it used to be.

Drug diversion sentences, allowed by such innovative ballot initiatives as California's Proposition 36, demonstrate the importance of giving judges the right to tailor their sentences for each case because drug addiction is a health issue, not a criminal one. Sending drug addicts, who tend to be notorious recidivists, to rehab hospitals instead of state prison is one way of reducing crime. The problem must be approached as one of rehabilitation rather than punishment.

Although *Saving America's* subtitle calls the U.S. a "Nation in Crisis," which it is, right thinking (as opposed to right-wing narrow-mindedness) will save us once again, just as it has in times of even greater crises like the Civil War and the Depression. America remains the greatest nation on earth, but it needs to change direction *now*, sooner rather than later, before the crises facing the nation become irreversibly unsolvable.

—the Honorable John Duran,
Mayor of West Hollywood, Calif.
June 11, 2007

INTRODUCTION

To America

I composed this tract to express my appreciation for this great country, which opened its doors to my family and me as immigrants in 1971. I was blessed to be able to raise my four children in America. I enjoyed a successful and gratifying career in the U.S. as a physician before retiring in 2007. I have achieved much more than I ever dreamt of.

In composing this work, I did not mean to criticize this country, but as an outsider before and an insider now, I have a unique perspective that can appreciate the problems which confront all Americans, especially the poor and the middle class.

During each election cycle, people get their hopes up, which quickly vanish after politicians take or resume office. This is a sad phenomenon I would like to see change, and this work offers many suggestions to accomplish that.

I like fairness in society. I don't advocate taking from the rich and giving to the poor by raising taxes. I'd rather see the rich stay rich, while the poor and the middle class become rich as well by improving education and healthcare, increasing wages, etc.

My goal is to save taxpayers' money and invest it in the U.S. for the benefit of the underprivileged. In general, I believe in less taxation, but if additional taxes provide tangible benefits to the people, I am in favor of them.

I believe in justice for all. Everyone should have the same opportunity for a good education and a good job through hard work as they climb the socio-economic ladder, but I don't believe in the Welfare system. It makes people dependent, lazy and a burden on the community.

People should live free of fear of street crime and domestic violence. America should act as a benevolent superpower and enjoy good relations with all the other nations of the world.

I believe people in power should serve their country and not abuse their power for personal gain.

I don't claim in this work to be perfect, but if I did criticize anyone, I was not judging him. I was judging the ones who are judging others, including the hypocrisy demonstrated by politicians and religious figures. I am neither conservative nor liberal, but a middle-of-the-road American.

My best wishes to all, and God bless America!

—Adel Shenouda, M.D., F.A.C.P.

June 11, 2007

CHAPTER ONE

Saving America From Congress and the President

The current crop of politicians in the United States Senate and Congress is doing nothing to help their constituents with the crisis-level problems facing the American people. Our national legislators are impotent and cannot pass desperately needed laws. The Republicans and Democrats block each other's legislation, and the President vetoes bills passed by Democrats.

Along with the threat of Presidential vetoes, filibusters in the Senate by the party out of power, the Republicans, are further blocking legislation that a slim Democratic majority in the Senate, as well as the American people, want to see enacted. Many bills creating affordable universal health insurance coverage, which polls show that 70 percent of the American public supports, languish in committee because Republicans oppose universal healthcare, and President Bush has repeatedly threatened to veto such legislation.

Tectonic Drift in D.C.

Also contributing to Congressional gridlock are powerful lobbyists representing major corporations such as drug and gun manufacturers. These special interests "buy" candidates by contributing to their reelection campaigns, and these candidates, who are returned to office at a rate of 80 percent because of gerrymandered voting districts, serve special interests at the expense of the constituents who elected them.

How Do We Unblock Gridlock?

The American people have been "brain-washed" into accepting the political platforms of one or the other two major parties in Congress. One platform or ideology is usually very bad, and the alternative platform is merely bad. One way to change this paradigm and reflect the will of the American people is through the establishment of a third and/or fourth party so no single party will have more than 40 percent of the vote in both houses of Congress, comparable to the multi-party system that exists in Germany, France, Israel and to a much less effective extent in the United Kingdom.

With a multiple-party system, two of the three or four parties will have to unite forces, as they frequently do in Israel's Knesset or parliament, and create a large enough voting bloc to overcome Senate filibusters (60 Senators required for that) and to override the inevitable Presidential vetoes (a two-thirds plus one vote of both houses are required for that).

Both the Democrats and Republicans are puppets who cater to their small liberal and conservative bases, respectively, which do not represent the political wishes of the majority of constituents of either major party. No one is acting on behalf of these majorities. In Germany, France and Israel as few as five members of the cabinet of the party in power can shift their allegiance to opposition parties, which causes the party in power to fall and new elections bring to office legislators who are not beholden to their previous party and can enact legislation which polls show the people want.

How to Create a Third or Fourth Party

That is a tall order which has been unsuccessfully tried in the past for more than a century, dating back to Teddy Roosevelt's feckless creation of the Bull Moose Party in 1912 after he lost the Republican presidential nomination to William Howard Taft, all the way up to the most recent attempt—Ralph Nader's resuscitation of the Green Party during the presidential election of 2000, which caused the defeat of the popularly elected candidate, Al Gore, and led to the Bush administration, the tragic war in Iraq, budget-busting deficit spending, decreases of government funding for programs that help the poor and the catastrophically ill, and perhaps the most tragic result of all—blocking funds for stem cell research, even though a majority of both Democratic and Republican legislators, as well as 70 percent of American voters, favor such research, with the exception of reactionary cranks like Rush Limbaugh and Bill O'Reilly.

This evaluation of the disastrous effects of the current administration's policies is not a fringe or partisan critique. Jimmy Carter has said, "I think as far as the adverse impact on the nation around the world, this Administration has been the worst in history." A White House spokesman responded that the ex-President is becoming "increasingly irrelevant." Senator Chuck Hagel, a Nebraska Republican, echoed Carter's criticism and called George W. Bush possibly the worst president in the history of the republic.

One of the goals of this work is to persuade the American people *not* to vote for Democratic or Republican candidates. Voters need to be oriented about the electoral process and how it perpetuates Congressional gridlock and the corruption of legislators by special interests. A year before the next national election, Americans need to be indoctrinated not to vote for the two major parties. Encourage independent candidates who are not associated with either of the two major parties or who left the Democrats or Republicans when they failed to be nominated for office representing their former parties, like Sen. Joe Lieberman and Pat Buchanan. They are not subservient to special interests or the bases of the Republican and Democratic parties.

The new entity might be called the American Independent Party. Since the creation of a political organization will require an infusion of cash, like-minded billionaires such as New York City Mayor and publishing magnate Michael Bloomberg, Bill Gates (the richest man in the world), Warren Buffett (the second richest in the U.S.), and Ross Perot, who have all denounced go-along politicians and politics as usual in the past, might be persuaded to jump start things by contributing to the new party and perhaps even volunteer to recruit candidates. A charismatic spokesman will also be a necessity for a successful effort, and an outspoken, anti-establishment figure like CNN anchor Lou Dobbs would make a perfect mouthpiece for it.

My recommendation to create a third party was anticipated during a May 2007 appearance on CBS' *Face the Nation*, when Republican Senator Chuck Hagel of Nebraska suggested the same thing—even sharing the top of the ticket with Mayor Bloomberg. "It's a great country to think about a New York boy and a Nebraska boy to be teamed up leading this nation," Hagel said on *Face the Nation*. Apparently, Hagel hadn't cleared his plan with Bloomberg before sharing it on TV. The next day, the Associated Press reported that Bloomberg rejected the idea out of hand and said, "I think [Hagel] was probably joking. He speaks his mind ... He's not happy with the same things that I'm not happy about."

Although the establishment of a third party might seem like the longest of long shots, some political scientists feel the current mood in the country makes starting a new party more feasible than in the past, since the last successful effort dates back to 1860, when Lincoln's four-year-old Republican Party won the presidency.

Professor Barry C. Burden at the University of Wisconsin-Madison said after Hagel's revelation, "There are some conditions in place that make it [now] seem more likely. One is the general sense of discontent in the electorate. It's partly the scandals and other issues that have plagued the Bush administration. The fact that the Iraq war doesn't have a resolution. The Democrats were swept into Congress [in 2006], but they're not solving those kinds of things."

Embryonic funding and a practical plan for this new party are already in place. The website Unity08.com plans to hold an on-line national primary in June 2008 to select a bipartisan ticket, which will require that the No. 1 and No. 2 candidates be of different parties to overcome partisan gridlock. So far, 60,000 delegates have signed up to participate in Unity08's primary with two million more delegates expected to jump on board. Contributions are already flowing in to the website.

Doug Bailey, a Republican consultant and a founder of Unity08, hopes the new party will attract centrists and diminish the ideological extremism of current presidential campaigns. "We anticipate, frankly, at that point [during the on-line June 2008 primary] a lot of people will be upset over the choices that were made, a lot of buyer's remorse. The country confronts too many serious issues at the very time it's political train has sort of left its tracks. You can't get anybody to work with anybody.... We can't afford four more years of that," Bailey said.

As the idea of a new party becomes more widely publicized, more Americans of lesser means will be persuaded to contribute to third-party candidates. To place a small party on the ballot will not cost the hundreds of millions of dollars currently being raised by presidential contenders from both major parties.

An even cheaper way to collect contributions for a third or fourth party is by getting free publicity by having independent candidates appear on Larry King's talk show, other CNN political programs—even Oprah might be receptive to this kind of free advertising. If she can turn books into massive best-sellers by having authors appear on her talk show, she can work the same magic and "sell" independent candidates. Buy my book. Vote for me. Same difference.

Another inexpensive method of raising initial funds for the new party's candidates is to hold local town hall meetings. Senatorial candidates will need to go to such meetings in every city in their state to debate and discuss the issues the American people really care about. Candidates for the House of Representatives will similarly attend town meetings in every city in their Congressional districts. Besides providing a platform for candidates to reveal their positions and game plans on vital issues, the town hall meetings can serve as a simple and practical way to raise funds in the form of contributions from voters who attend these town meetings. Local TV stations or PBS should also provide free airtime to all candidates, especially third party candidates who lack the funding of major parties. Regardless of whether they represent the two current major parties or the new independent party, all candidates should receive the same amount of money raised by town hall meetings, and all should get equal amounts of free TV air-time.

Voters can be encouraged to contribute at these town hall meetings by being reminded that the major party candidates get their money from special interests—corporations who pass on the cost of campaign spending to the consumer by raising the cost of the products they manufacture or sell. The American people should know that they are the ultimate sponsors of major party candidates because the cost of corporate campaign funding shows up at the cash register, where they pay extra for their purchases.

The most important goal of the independent party will be to prevent either the Republicans or Democrats from controlling more than 40 percent of the two houses of Congress, overcoming gridlock, corporate corruption and White House vetoes. Elected members of the new party will bring fresh blood to our stagnant legislatures—representatives of the people who are not controlled by corporate lobbies and will not follow like sheep the demands of the masters of the Republican and Democratic parties.

Another way to bring fresh blood to Washington is to set term-limits and bring in newcomers with new ideas, who will enact well-crafted legislation which the Supreme Court will be prevented from overturning as it has in the past because the legislation with meet Constitutional requirements. Incumbents' decades in power lead to a sense of entitlement, taking for granted (i.e., ignoring) the will of constituents, with metastasizing variations on corruption like bribery and sex scandals. Senate incumbents should not be allowed to remain in office for more than two terms or 12 years. Incumbents in the House of Representatives should be kicked out after four terms or eight years.

While we will lose many long-serving incumbents like Congressman Henry Waxman of California and Senator Christopher Dodd of Connecticut who have developed impressive expertise in enacting legislation after decades in office, too many incumbents are merely time-servers who after 25 years have no fresh ideas, prefer the feckless status quo and share the same mentality of not rocking the boat. Go along to get along. To these dinosaur incumbents, I would say, "Thank you and have a prosperous and fulfilling retirement. Good-bye."

Although term limits will cause the loss of experts like Waxman and Dodd, the loss will not be irrecoverable. New members of Congress during their first term will observe and learn the complexities of the legislative process. During their second—and final—term, they will become competent and well-trained chairmen of Senate and Congressional committees and subcommittees.

Six Years and You're Out

Term-limits should not be forced on the Federal legislative branch alone. One way to make the President a more effective administrator and less a politician is to mandate a single, six-year term for the presidency, as Mexico already does.

With the current situation that allows the president to serve two four-year terms, during his first term, he spends two to three years focusing on partisan political issues, excessively concentrating on getting reelected to a second term, which influences—often to ill effect—many of his decisions as Chief Executive. President Clinton didn't get involved with the Palestinian-Israeli debacle until his second term.

Suicidally, President Jimmy Carter, probably the most apolitical President of our times, didn't wait for a second term and treated Israel and the Palestinians even-handedly, which probably was a factor in his failed second presidential bid, although the primary reason for his loss was the state of the economy—as measured by the "misery index," which combined the rate of inflation with the rate of unemployment to gauge just how "miserable" American voters were.

As Presidential contender Ronald Reagan during the 1980 Presidential campaign asked to great effect, "Are you better off now than you were four years ago?" With inflation running at 14 percent and unemployment at 11 percent in 1980, the answer was a resounding "NO!" and reinforced in voters' minds just how dissatisfied they were with the Carter administration. Reagan, who in August 1980 had been trailing Carter by 33 percentage points, ended up winning with one of the biggest landslides in presidential electoral history.

To increase his reelection chances and gain friends in Congress to support his bid for a second term, the President spends too much time flying all over the country, especially during mid-term elections, delivering speeches in favor of his Congressional allies seeking reelection. This reduces the time he can spend doing the job he was elected to do—govern the country. Decreasing the number of his campaign flights on Air Force One with administration officials, secret service agents and a full media contingent in tow will save taxpayer and campaign money.

When the President makes campaign flights unrelated to his Presidential duties, he does pay airfare, but it's a fraction of the actual cost of flying such a mob of hangers-on, plus he gets the money to finance his flights from special interests, thus furthering his dependence on these groups, which already have too much influence over the President and Congress.

If and when the President is reelected, during his second, lame-duck term, he tends to be less focused on campaigning for political friends because he no longer needs their help to get reelected. Congress, after FDR overstayed his welcome in the White House during four terms, enacted legislation during the Truman administration limiting the President to two.

But while the President is able to concentrate less on political considerations, his second-term administration will experience "executive fatigue," and he will not perform well. Also, by the time his second term begins, he will have made so many enemies among the opposition party in Congress, that it will be harder for him to reach compromises with his opponents and enact legislation. Proof of this enmity is that the number of Presidential vetoes typically increases during a second term compared to the first.

I would go so far as to make it illegal for the President to campaign for the election and reelection of his political cronies so he can concentrate 100 percent on serving the people's non-partisan interests. He should be the President of all Americans during his single six years in office, not just the representative of his party.

After he leaves office, he, of course, should be allowed to campaign for political friends as much as he wants. Despite his scandalous Presidency, Bill Clinton remains enormously popular and his speeches for political candidates are much sought-after prizes. Proof of his popularity is that he often charges $200,000 a pop to speak to political and corporate organizations.

Another benefit of a single-term presidency is that the President will not be afraid of crossing members of his own party or alienating special interests, whose campaign contributions won't be needed for a second term.

Voters are not blameless for keeping their representatives marinating in power for decades. Americans often prefer to vote for incumbents of 20 to 30 years' duration even when their representatives are so old they develop Alzheimer's disease because the longer politicians stay in office, the more power they accumulate, which allows them to deliver pork barrel legislation like earmarks to their Congressional districts and states. Senator Strom Thurmond remained in office for close to 50 years, only departing the chamber shortly before his death at age 101.

CHAPTER TWO

Saving America From Special Interests

Another way to break the chokehold the two major parties currently exercise over the national government is to forbid candidates from rejecting matching government funding of their campaigns because they know they can raise much, much more money from special interests. All campaigns for the legislature and the president should be funded solely by the government. During an election year, American taxpayers should be required to contribute a nominal one half of one percent of their income to fund campaigns of all candidates.

They can pay this amount at the same time they pay their federal income taxes. Currently taxpayers can opt to contribute $5 to campaigns, but the government gives this money exclusively to members of the two major parties, one of the reasons Ralph Nader revived the Green Party in 2000 so his candidates could partake of government largesse. Unfortunately, to receive government funds, each party has to score at least five percent of the vote to be funded for the next election, and Nader, while successfully denying Al Gore the presidency, failed to get more than two and a half percent of the vote, and his party did not become eligible for government funding. Karma.

With the current two-party system, incumbents would never enact legislation that would forbid them from rejecting government funding for their campaigns and eliminate contributions from special interests because they can raise so much more money on their own compared to what the government is willing to contribute. But if third-party candidates are elected, they can push through laws that will force major party candidates to accept matching government funds and turn away corporate donations. These third-party candidates can also legislate a limit to the amount of money that can be spent on campaigns to a figure much lower than the current staggering average cost of $200 million per presidential candidate. Experts predict that the 2008 race for the presidency will be the most expensive in history, totaling $1 billion.

Another way of pressuring incumbents to accept government funding and reject campaign contributions from special interests is to publicize exactly how much money incumbents receive from special interests. The skill and expertise of investigative journalists can reveal how legislators enact laws that benefit their corporate benefactors. The identity of these special interests and their financial contributions to favored candidates is already matter of public record but not aggressively disseminated. The job of third-party activists will be to publicize to whom and how much money is donated by fat cats. The American people should "buy" candidates, not special interest groups whose "interests" are often not in the best interest of the American people.

Right now, there are many qualified independent candidates who can run for office, but they usually lack the money to gain national exposure through expensive radio and TV commercials. Government funding of these competent and incorruptible politicians would level the playing field and help establish a third and/or fourth party.

Another way to eliminate the corrupting influence of special interests who pay the obscene amounts needed to win elections is to limit the campaign season to six months, as they do in European and other industrialized countries, instead of the current interminable U.S. presidential campaigns which drag on for two years and cause voter burnout and cynicism. (The very next day after President Bush was first elected to office in

2000, newspapers were already handicapping the prospects of presidential candidates in the 2004 election!)

A shorter campaign season will naturally result in less contributions by corporate lobbyists. Another reason for a mandated six-month campaign season is that the current two-year period of running for office distracts legislators from their real job, which is enacting legislation the American people have shown they want, such as affordable health insurance for every citizen, gun control, crime reduction and more funding for public schools.

Cheaper campaigns will also lessen the financial influence of another special interest group, the Christian Evangelical right, which is obsessed with non-religious issues that polls show the American people don't really have any interest in, such as illegalizing abortion and banning gay marriage.

When Mary Cheney, the lesbian daughter of the Vice President, gave birth to a baby boy in May 2007, it was red meat to the Christian ultra right. Stephen Bennett, the founder of Stephen Bennett Ministries, an organization that tries to "convert" gays and turn them straight, called Mary's baby a "tragedy" and deplored the White House's official website featuring a photo of the proud grandparents Dick and Lynne Cheney holding their new grandson, Samuel David.

Bennett blogged on the WorldNetDaily.com website in June 2007, "I guess we can tragically … say both the White House and the Bush Administration have officially recognized the sinful sexual unions of homosexuals, as well as embraced the tragedy of the social experiment of homosexual parenting…. I say shame on the White House, shame on the president and shame on the vice president for allowing such a caption to be 'officially' added onto the White House website and such a beautiful photo of two happy grandparents and their new grandchild." The photo's caption sounded innocent enough and simply said, "… [Samuel David's] parents are the Cheneys' daughter Mary, and her partner, Heather Poe. White House photo by David Bohrer."

If you're not pregnant or gay, you don't care about abortion or whether or not two gay men or women can exchange wedding rings and register their silverware patterns at Neiman Marcus. The ideological extremism of religious groups distracts legislators from issues the American people do care about—issues which will help all Americans. The theology of Evangelicals, which they try to masquerade as political issues, is of no interest to mainstream citizens; it's just ideological atavism.

Religious fundamentalists are more interested in politics than religion. They use hot-button issues like abortion and gay rights to promote or defeat political candidates. We never hear them talk about genuine moral issues, like ending the war in Iraq, Federal funding for embryonic stem cell research or taking guns out of the hands of mentally ill mass murderers like the paranoid schizophrenic who gunned down 32 fellow students at Virginia Tech in April 2007.

One of our most prominent Christian fundamentalist televangelists once insisted that war is morally justifiable because God is pro-war! He had apparently been reading too much of the Old Testament with its vengeful deity who ordered Joshua to slay all the Canaanite inhabitants of Jericho, including women and children, and who tormented Job for no apparent reason other than sadism.

Fundamentalists ignore social issues like poverty, healthcare and education. They never promote legislation which religion instructs us will improve the lives of Americans. These religious leaders lead Ivory Tower lives, ensconced in palatial mansions with their private jets and their own television networks. They condemn the moral behavior of others while often hiding their own malfeasance such as sex scandals and money laundering. They are aggressively judgmental, ignoring Jesus' admonition, "Let ye among you without sin cast the first stone." Televangelists who smoke methamphetamine with male prostitutes and Bible Belt Congressmen who send White House pages sexually explicit emails and Instant Messages should *not* be casting stones at other alleged moral transgressors.

The Evangelical right holds power completely out of proportion to their actual numbers, which represent only a tiny fraction of the Republican electorate. What the Christian fundamentalists do have is a huge war chest to buy influence among legislators. One way to circumvent their financial advantage is to educate Americans not to vote for candidates backed by special interests like Evangelicals. Unfortunately, voters need a lot of "education" to counter their current indifference to this issue. "Polls only show that five percent of the public feel [campaign finance reform] is important," Georgetown University historian Michael Kazin said. "It is just too complicated."

If the Christian right is promoting candidate X, let the American people know so they can vote for candidate Y. Investigative reporters and political reform activists should expose candidates supported by these special interests and publicize exactly how much money these interests contribute to each candidate beholden to their fundamentalist masters. Federal law already requires such public disclosures, but they get less attention from the media than Alec Baldwin's telephone etiquette.

Proof of the lack of interest in these tangential issues promoted by the Evangelical right and other special interests is the astoundingly successful candidacy of former New York City mayor Rudy Giuliani. Although he is a member of the conservative Republican party, he has remained largely faithful to his liberal past as the former chief executive of a liberal city, unlike ideological turncoats such as former Massachusetts governor and closet liberal Mitt Romney, who has abandoned his life-long liberal views and proclaimed himself a born-again conservative, to the point of trying to appeal to NRA supporters by claiming that he is an avid hunter even though he has gone hunting a grand total of two times. Romney lamely insists his credentials as a hunter are valid because, as he says, "I've been shooting little varmints all my life."

Romney seems unable to escape his pro-choice rights past which has come back to haunt him. Speaking at a banquet organized by Massachusetts Citizens for Life, on May 10, 2007, he said, "Human life has a profound dignity.... And so I publicly acknowledged my error, and joined with you to promote the sanctity of human life." Pro-choice advocates mocked Romney's new born-again pro-life posturing by picketing the dinner wearing flip-flop shoes to symbolize his flip-flopping on the issue.

Romney's *faux* reincarnation as a Great White Hunter to court NRA support is reminiscent of 1988 presidential candidate Michael Dukakis' attempt to establish military cred by riding around with his head poking out of a tank wearing an ill-fitting helmet which led pundits to lampoon him as resembling Michael Schultz' Snoopy.

By contrast, Giuliani has maintained his huge lead in the polls that rank Republican presidential candidates by sticking to his guns, supporting gay rights, protecting a woman's right to choose and calling for more rigorous gun control—all positions that are anathema to the Republican base. Giuliani's front-runner position proves that he is addressing the needs and concerns of the American people, not the fringe obsessions of ultra-conservatives who are able to deny a candidate a primary win but don't have the power to decide a presidential election.

Voters, including moderate Republicans, don't care that Giuliani was unfaithful to his second wife, moved in with two gay guys and their poodle after he left Mrs. No. 2 in the mayor's official residence Gracie Mansion. Voters also seem indifferent to other Giuliani outrages, like telling the same second missus that he was divorcing her—not to face to face but during a press conference!

But most amazingly of all, in a country that still harbors a great deal of subterranean homophobia, no one seems to object to Giuliani occasionally putting on a dress, wig and makeup and performing at gala charity fundraisers, although as the 2008 presidential election campaign heats up and gets even nastier than now, we can expect to see endless replays on television of videotape of the former mayor camping it up in drag. Such startling images already crop up on the airwaves, yet fail to put a dent in Giuliani's front-runner status.

Some religious conservatives, unlike a plurality of their peers who pick Giuliani as their top choice for president, aren't willing to give Giuliani a pass on his past. Perhaps out of despair and desperation because he's at the back of the pack of presidential hopefuls, former Arkansas Governor Mike Huckabee, referring to Giuliani's irregular mating habits and conservative voters' tolerance of them, said, "It would a complete loss of credibility for Christian evangelical leaders to suddenly say, With Republicans, we're going to have a new set of rules. It applied to Bill Clinton, but won't apply to anyone else." Huckabee has not read the polls.

A former Baptist minister, Huckabee believes that personal and professional behavior are not inseparable and referring to Giuliani's irregular past resorted to this *non-sequitur*: "If I fail to keep the promises I make to the people closest to me, then I'm not sure how reliable I'm going to be in keeping promises to total strangers who vote for me."

Benjamin Ginsberg, director of the Center for the Study of American Government at Johns Hopkins, offers a compelling theory for Giuliani's Teflon immunity from his Don Juan past. "We're in the post-Clinton era. People have become more tolerant of personal foibles. The only way a candidate can be really hurt by revelations now is to deny. They get killed by the lies and deceptions." Giuliani doesn't hide or deny his curious concept of marital fidelity or lack thereof. As legions have already pointed out, perjury, not fellatio by a White House intern, got Clinton impeached ... and disbarred from the practice of law for five years.

Denial and lies are not only fatal to political careers, they harm all people in the public eye. After a male prostitute outed televangelist Ted Haggard and claimed they shared a methamphetamine-filled pipe, Haggard confessed to the ministers who sit on the board of his church that the hustler had told the truth. His board forgave him, and after a traditional period of repentance, voted to let him return to his ministry. Then, while Haggard was pulling out of his driveway, he was ambushed by a TV camera crew, and a reporter asked him about the prostitute's revelations. Haggard, looking, well, haggard, nervous and caught off-guard, lied, claiming he just received a massage from the hustler and never smoked methamphetamine with his hired companion.

This apparently contradicted what he had told his board of ministers, and after they got a look at the videotape of his ambush interview, the ministers announced that while they had been willing to forgive Haggard for his sexual and narcotics transgressions, since he lied to the TV reporter, he would never be allowed back into the mega-church he had founded. Haggard had so disenchanted his board that it didn't help when later, the male prostitute, Mike Jones, failed a lie detector test. To quote the cliché, honesty is the best policy no matter how embarrassing the revelation.

Giuliani's integrity and fidelity to his ideological past have not only prevented him from losing the support of the Christian right, he leads the pack among such voters, who despise yet ignore his left-leaning philosophy. A *Los Angeles Times* poll conducted in April 2007 revealed that he remains the No. 1 favorite nationwide among white conservative Christians who comprise the Republican base.

Twenty-six percent of these voters prefers Giuliani, double the number who favor increasingly right-wing Republican presidential candidates Senator John McCain and former Governor Mitt Romney.

Archconservatives may have to hold their noses when they vote for a candidate like Giuliani who represents so much of what they loathe ideologically, but some of Giuliani's other attributes keep them in his corner. Iowa voter Mike Brown abhors Giuliani's pro-choice position among others, but during his state's crucial caucuses, which take place earliest in the presidential primary and often anoint the front-runner, Brown will swallow hard and vote for the former mayor of New York City.

Brown told the *Los Angeles Times* in April 2007, "You want someone who's demonstrated character." A city employee of Pella, Iowa, Brown disregards Giuliani's liberal baggage and wants him to become the next president because of the take-charge leadership the candidate demonstrated as New York's chief executive after the 9/11 attacks. Brown said, "Just being able to remain calm, dispatch the people, handle the situation—those are things I really find favorable."

Another reaction to 9/11, a generalized terror of Islamic terrorists, also prompts the Christian right to favor the leftist candidate over his conservative competitors. Dennis J. Goldford, who teaches political science at Drake University in Des Moines, Iowa, theorizes that religious fundamentalists believe America is engaged in a "massive, titanic ideological struggle with radical Islam. Religious conservatives," Goldford told the *Los Angeles Times*, "have come to see radical Islam as the dominant issue of the age to the point that for some of them—not all—this eclipses things like abortion, taxes and homosexuality." Paranoia about Muslim extremists has become the 21st century equivalent of the 20th century West's dread of the

Soviet bogeyman's expansionism in Southeast Asia, Latin America and Africa.

Other right-leaning voters support Giuliani despite his knee-jerk liberal positions for more practical reasons that have nothing to do with political ideology and everything to do with *Realpolitik*. Giuliani, they believe, and polls bear them out, is the only Republican who can win the general election in November 2008. Conservative Joy Milby, another resident of Pella, Iowa, said, "We have some differences, but he's electable."

Voters like Milby are certain that the other lead contenders, such as Senator John McCain, with his self-sabotaging support of President Bush's troop surge in Baghdad and ex-governor Mitt Romney's suspicious flip-flopping from liberal to conservative that seems to turn off both ends of the political spectrum, don't have a prayer at becoming our 44th Commander in Chief.

Despite the tolerance and acceptance of conservatives, Giuliani has not remained 100 percent ideologically pure and has moved rightward on several issues. He applauded the April 2007 decision of the U.S. Supreme Court to ban so-called "partial birth abortions," which during the third trimester involves partially exposing the fetus outside its mother's vaginal cavity, then either crushing the fetus' skull or vacuuming its brain out, even though as recently as 1997 Giuliani supported the procedure.

The former mayor's promise to appoint Supreme Court Justices in the mold of Paleolithic conservatives like Antonin Scalia sounds as though he has fallen through Alice's Looking Glass, or as another Paleolithic conservative, Pat Buchanan, said in a May 11, 2007, syndicated column, "Rudy's pro-choice, pro-Scalia stance seems intellectually incoherent and politically inexplicable."

Despite his lead in the polls, Giuliani appears to be tortured by his pro-abortion rights position and some of his statements on the matter have been contradictory—or as the *Los Angeles Times* described them, "rhetorical contortions." The *bête noire* of the Christian right and Giuliani's Achilles Heel, the abortion issue has led him to say things that make the term "flip-flopping" seem like rock solid conviction such as his assertion that it would be "OK" if Roe Vs. Wade—the 1973 Supreme Court decision that enshrined a woman's right to choose—were overturned, and "OK" if it were upheld.

An editorial in the conservative *Wall Street Journal* on May 11, 2007, scolded all Republican candidates and warned them to continue debating abortion at their own electoral peril: "An abortion fight will make the party seem irrelevant to the main voter concerns, or captive to its litmus test interests."

On another occasion, Giuliani adopted the classic liberal position on abortion rights espoused by Hillary Clinton and John Kerry, *et al.*, when he made the by now clichéd statement in a speech to hundreds of Christian conservatives at Houston Baptist University, calling abortion "morally wrong" but maintained his belief that women should have "the right to make that choice." This kind of equivocation does not mollify the Christian right.

Republicans make a strategic mistake when they ignore the issue of abortion rights or worse, try to ban the procedure. Between 1973, the year the Supreme Court's Roe vs. Wade decision virtually gave women the right to abortion on demand, and 2002, more than 42 million legal abortions were performed, according to the Alan Guttmacher Institute, a Washington, D.C.-based think tank that promotes sexual and reproductive health. In 2002, the most recent year for which statistics are available, 1.29 million abortions took place. Twenty-four percent of all pregnancies end in abortion, Guttmacher reported. Throw in the relatives and loved ones of the 42 million who opted for terminating their pregnancies over the past three decades, and you have a huge constituency that will vote against any candidate who wants to overturn Roe vs. Wade or enact a Constitutional amendment outlawing a woman's right to choose.

Personally, I have no position on the abortion issue—for or against. A Gallup Poll in 2003 reported that a large majority of voters, over 60 percent, do not want the Supreme Court to overturn Roe vs. Wade. Americans care about genuinely important issues like healthcare, embryonic stem cell research, crime reduction, education reform, poverty, and safety from domestic terrorist attacks. Rudy Giuliani's position at the top of the polls is due to his focus on these issues rather than abortion or gay marriage. Only special interest groups like the Evangelical right are obsessed with abortion and gay rights. As surveys show, any candidate who focuses on those tangential issues or flip-flops will find himself at the back of the pack, e.g., ex-governors Mike Huckabee and Mitt Romney.

Despite his double-digit lead over all other candidates, Giuliani has tried to have it both ways on issues that obsess the conservative base of his party. He continues to defend New York gun control laws while maintaining that he believes in "the personal right to bear arms." Like most politicians, left or right, Giuliani is not willing to commit electoral suicide by approving gay marriage, but he still alienates his base by supporting gay rights, including gay unions, which represent gay marriage in all but name only. (No wedding cake or rings, but spousal benefits like insurance coverage and inheritance rights, etc.)

While campaigning in Alabama in 2007, Giuliani switched another position and said individual states should be allowed to decide whether or not to fly the Confederate flag from statehouse capitols. He has also abandoned his earlier support of a national ban on handguns and now wants each state to formulate its own firearm legislation.

Yet another example of Giuliani's glacial creep toward the right is the evolution of his position on U.S. immigration policy. During his mayoralty, he fought Washington's unbelievably cruel efforts to limit illegal immigrants' access to public hospitals and deny their children a free education. He based his stance on practical rather than legalistic arguments. Back then, he said, "The reality is that they are here, and they are going to remain here." But for his current national audience, he has become even more reactionary than President Bush and opposes Bush's proposal to grant undocumented workers amnesty. This is a startling 180-degree turn from his tenure as mayor of New York when he proposed spending $12 million to create a program that would help immigrants gain U.S. citizenship. By 2007, he was demanding penalties for illegal immigrants and called for their return to Mexico or other countries while they pursued legal reentry to the United States.

Then there's the puzzling case of Senator John McCain, a puzzling and contradictory combination of political expediency and just the opposite—

self-sabotaging honesty backing unpopular issues that seem unwise if not downright suicidal for someone who seeks the top job in 2008. In the expediency column is his current failure to bring up campaign finance reform, the issue which almost allowed him to snatch the presidential nomination away from George Bush early in the 2000 race. He never addresses the subject during the 2008 campaign. That could be due to expediency. The Senator may have read polls that show that only five percent of voters care about campaign financing reform because the issue is simply too complicated and not "sexy" enough like partial-birth abortions or stopping lesbians from donning bridal wear.

Another expedient *volte-face* is his position on the Confederate flag. In 2000, during a speech in the Deep South, he had the courage to denounce flying the Stars and Bars as a "symbol of racism and poverty." Jump cut to 2007, in the same state, South Carolina, when reporters asked him how he felt about participants at a political rally he was attending who were waving the flag of the Old South, he said, "Welcome to South Carolina. It's a free country."

At the opposite end of the strategy spectrum, his self-sabotaging honesty has surfaced in at least two issues where he supports his former nemesis-in-chief, George Bush. A one-time critic of Bush's increase in tax cuts for the super rich who once said he could not vote for them "in good conscience," by 2007 he was defending these tax breaks by explaining that ending the cuts would amount to a "tax increase." Favoring the rich is not an effective way to court the middle class vote, and the tax cuts have contributed to Bush's approval rating falling to the mid-30 percent range during his last two years in office. That kind of unpopularity is contagious and may explain why Rudy Giuliani leads McCain by double-digits in polls conducted in 2007.

McCain's stance on abortion appears to depend on geographical location. In conservative South Carolina, he denounced abortion rights. In liberal New Hampshire, he kept mum on the hot-button issue.

Another candidate with an even squeakier clean reputation as a campaign finance reform purist is Democratic hopeful Barack Obama. But in the spring of 2007, the *Los Angeles Times* ran a front-page story "outing"

Obama as a closet pawn of fat cat contributors with an impressive knack for political sophistry that might have made a Jesuit casuist in 18th century France blush. The Senator from Illinois performed a bit of verbal gymnastics when he pledged early in his campaign to reject money from *Washington* lobbyists. His platform website says he will not accept funding by "federal lobbyists" and crowed that in the spring of 2007 he virtuously returned $43,000 of lobby money.

His Internet appeals for funding boast a holier-and-less-greed-ier-than-thou, above-the-grubby-fray philosophy by asserting, "It may sound strange for a presidential candidate to launch a fundraising drive that isn't about dollars. But our democracy shouldn't be about money, and it's time our campaigns weren't either."

That is dead-on correct, but Obama doesn't practice what he electronically preaches. What his website has conveniently neglected to add was that he does accept donations from lawyers whose partners are lobbyists. As the *Times'* article also reported without putting a dent in Obama's rock-star like popularity, he will also accept contributions from lobbyists who aren't based in Washington. State-based lobbyists are welcome to fill Obama's coffers. "Clearly, the distinction [between federal and state lobbyists] is not that significant," said Stephen Weissman of the Campaign Finance Institute, a nonpartisan think tank that studies the electoral process.

Weissman may be too generous when he calls the distinction insignificant since a more accurate term might be irrelevant. "He gets an asterisk that says he is trying to be different, but overall, the same wealthy interests are funding his campaign as are funding other candidates, whether or not they are [technically] lobbyists," Weissman added. Obama's moral relativism when it comes to distinguishing between non-lobbying lawyers and lobbyists outside the Beltway has dramatically paid off. His massive war chest made national headlines when it was reported that in the first quarter of 2007, Obama raked in $27 million, almost the same amount as front-runner Hillary Clinton. And by spring of 2007, Clinton's once double-digit lead in the polls over Obama had shrunk to a statistically insignificant two percentage points.

During the first three months of 2007, Obama's election committee reported that he received money from 104,000 supporters, double the number as Clinton, which implies that he receives much smaller amounts from individual donors in order to match Clinton's haul. But the Campaign Finance Institute reported that Obama nevertheless got 68 percent of his funding from people contributing $1,000 or more each, a troubling percentage for advocates of ending non-government campaign financing, but still much lower than Clinton's comparable 86 percent of similar-sized donations.

Even massive assistance from lawyers who aren't lobbyists or from non-Washington-based lobbyists is welcome by Obama's election committee. The blue chip law firm of Alston & Bird gave the candidate $33,000 in early 2007, but the money came from partners in the firm who are not registered as lobbyists while other partners are. And the firm's headquarters are located in Atlanta, although it does have a Washington branch, and it does hire lobbyists, but they don't contribute to Obama's war chest. While the Senator rejects money from Washington-based lobbyists, he does accept contributions from Washington firms that employ lobbyists.

In the first three months of 2007, Obama contributors Goldman Sachs and Citigroup, two major investment houses that have legislation under consideration by Congress, paid lobbyists $4.6 million in 2006 to influence Washington lawmakers.

The Obama campaign has also accepted donations from such unsavory outfits like nuclear power plant owners. The nation's largest, the Exelon Corp., spent half a million dollars on federal legislators in 2006. Obama didn't take any money from Exelon's Washington-based lobbyists in keeping with his pledge to refuse assistance from the Beltway lobbying fraternity, but he did accept thousands of dollars from Springfield, Illinois-based lobbyists John P. Novak and James Monk, who are employed by a trade association that represents an Exelon-subsidiary, Commonwealth Edison. Other lobbying firms with headquarters outside the nation's capital who represent AT&T, United Airlines, the Recording Industry of America, trial attorneys, insurance companies, fast-food chains, sugar cane growers, and the Florida-based law firm of Akerman Senterfitt, whose website shamelessly boasts that it enjoys "an enviable level access" to members of Congress.

In perhaps an even sleazier financial association, on May 2, 2007, the Illinois Senator attended a pricey $2,300—per-person breakfast—a lot of money for ham and eggs but a bargain for the influence that kind of money can buy—which was hosted by 22 attorneys who are not registered Washington lobbyists but three of whom have worked as lobbyists in the past and are partners in a law firm that has in-house as well as outside lobbyists who deal with Congress.

One of the lawyers who hosted the May breakfast has represented polluters who have fought off lawsuits demanding they perform toxic waste cleanups and other groups that oppose early retirement legislation, all of which they admit on their websites. Other lawyers who hosted the breakfast fundraiser for Obama have represented defense contractors, energy producers, healthcare insurance companies, drug makers and the tobacco industry.

Obama's semantical hair-splitting distinctions between federal and state-based lobbyists does not impress his critics. Political scientist Bruce Cain, director of the University of California's Washington Center, said, "If you cannot be completely pure, is it worth it to be partially pure? That seems to be debatable." It's a debate that must be taken up by the American public because it is not being seriously considered by most of its representatives in the nation's capital.

Like her closest rival, Barack Obama, Hillary Clinton has also been tainted by an association with one of her biggest donors, billionaire TV producer and executive Haim Saban. Since 1999, the Egyptian-born Israeli and American citizen has contributed $40,400 to Clinton's campaign coffers. The Hollywood-based mogul loves both Clintons and has donated $5 million to Bill Clinton's presidential library in Little Rock, Arkansas, and loaned the project another $10 million. The library repaid the loan, but Saban forgave $2.4 million in interest. Although a Senate committee in 2007 was investigating allegations that Saban evaded paying $300 million in taxes on a $1.5 billion capital gain, both Clintons have refused to return Saban's contributions, unlike Senator John McCain, co-author of the 2002 McCain-Feingold campaign finance reform law, who in 2006 returned a $20,000 contribution from Texas software billionaire brothers, Sam and Charles J. Wyly, Jr., to McCain's presidential race after a Senate committee investigated them for allegedly creating 58 overseas trusts and corporate shells which allowed them to evade taxes on $190 million in corporate compensation. McCain also canceled the brothers' participation in a 2006 Dallas fundraiser, at which time a campaign spokesman said the Arizona Senator returns all contributions from anyone under investigation.

During his 2000 run for the presidency, then Vice President Al Gore demonstrated a less egregious form of campaign hypocrisy when he presented himself as a champion of the poor, which he is, and a class enemy of the very rich, which in reality he is not. He frequently bashed the wealthy and promised he would not cut their taxes. Post-election surveys estimated that he lost between one and two percent of the vote of affluent voters, Democrats who likely would have voted for him if he hadn't alienated them by deploring their privileged, under taxed existence.

Gore's hypocrisy, while not on a scale of Barack Obama's acceptance of special interest money or Mitt Romney's born-again conservatism, derived from the fact that he had been one of the richest members of the Senate while condemning his financial peers, and it didn't help his credibility when it was revealed that he lived in a luxe 10,000-square-foot mansion in his home state of Tennessee. I don't blame him for being rich or that he lives in a palace, but it is good for everyone to prosper in America. He masqueraded as an enemy of the rich while being one of them.

2008 presidential contender John Edwards also presents himself as a populist representative of the working class despite a personal fortune estimated at $25 million accumulated during his years as a personal injury (read ambulance-chasing) attorney. In fact, he's put himself forward as an expert on the predicament of the poor with the publication of his book *Ending Poverty in America: How to Restore the American Dream.*

His luxurious lifestyle was exposed and ridiculed when the media reported that he once spent $400 on a haircut, which shockingly was paid for with campaign money, and when that information leaked out, he reimbursed his campaign. Edwards' haircut easily topped Bill Clinton's record for shelling out $200 for a trim and blow-dry. Edwards himself admitted his high-priced trip to the barber was a strategic blunder. "It was just a mistake," he said. "It was a ridiculous amount to pay for a haircut.... [But] I don't think it has had any lasting impact." Or as the Los Angeles Times described his *faux pas*, it was "an unusual stumble for a candidate attuned to the power of symbols in politics." To reestablish his reputation as the Robin Hood of presidential politics, in the same interview in which he apologized for his extravagant haircut, he reminded readers that his father was a humble mill worker and Edwards himself did manual labor during summer breaks in college. He doesn't remind readers that he lives in a 28,000-square-foot mansion on a 100-acre estate.

As F. Scott Fitzgerald never said, the rich *are* different from you and me. Of course, there's no inherent contradiction in being mega-rich while advocating increased aid to the poor. Hollywood is packed with "limousine liberals" like Steven Spielberg and David Geffen, who are never taken to task for their multi-billion dollar fortunes while championing left-wing causes. But for credibility reasons, it's probably best not to ape the lavish *nouveau riche* spending style of tycoons like the imprisoned ex-Tyco CEO Dennis Kozlowski, who was barbecued by the media for paying $6,000 for a shower curtain and a $2 million birthday party for his wife on the Italian island of Sardinia using company funds.

Moreover, if even Mr. Clean avatars like Barack Obama can be influenced (cynics might say corrupted) by crypto-lobbyists such as the Atlanta law firm and companies that refuse to clean up the toxic waste they dump, the necessity of mandatory, not voluntary, rejection of special interest contributions is all the more urgent.

The beauty of a third and/or fourth party is that it will replicate the characteristics of any buyer-seller negotiation that takes place in the business world. On specific issues, the third party will collaborate with members of one of the two major parties. In the business world, when two corporations want to make a deal to buy or sell anything, they sit together, agree to compromises and at the end of negotiations they come up with a deal. The same process will work for enacting compromise legislation that will have enough support to halt filibusters and override presidential vetoes.

Truly independent third-party legislators will provide an antidote to the shocking bias demonstrated by major party members of both Houses when they sit on committees and subcommittees that investigate malfeasance by government officials. One egregious example of this bias was displayed by Senator Orrin Hatch of Utah during his 1987 "interrogation" of Col. Oliver North at the height of the Iran-Contra scandal. Instead of trying to ferret out the truth about North's participation in illegal activities, which resulted in a felony conviction later overturned on a technicality, Hatch used his platform on the investigative committee to praise North as an American hero while most Americans were condemning his felonious behavior.

Hatch actually seemed to be bragging about North rather than questioning or critiquing him. Twenty years later, Hatch was at it again and had become an apologist for U.S. Attorney General Alberto R. Gonzales, supporting Gonzales' decision to fire eight U.S. attorneys or Federal prosecutors in contrast to fellow Republican Senator Arlen Specter who criticized the Attorney General's politicization of the prosecutors' terminations. As Yogi Berra said, "It's *deja vu* all over again." Covering up or dismissing the seriousness of government malefactors does a disservice to the American people who want the truth, not dissembling.

Bias is not the inevitable *modus operandi* of major party legislators. During hearings on the Watergate scandal in 1975, Senator Howard Baker of Tennessee took to task a member of his own party, President Nixon, asking pointed questions in order to expose the participation of White House operatives in the Watergate break-in and the ensuing cover-up by top Nixon advisors Bob Haldeman and John D. Erlichman.

CHAPTER THREE
Saving America From the Ultra Right Wing

The increasingly conservative composition of the U.S. Supreme Court, which does not reflect the will of the majority of American citizens on issues like abortion and gun control, can also be neutralized by a national referendum. It is next to impossible to "reform" the Supreme Court which has consistently overturned as unconstitutional term-limits for incumbents and has been nibbling away at Roe vs. Wade, the 1973 Supreme Court decision that gave women the right to abortion on demand. In April 2007, the court illegalized so-called "partial birth abortions," a decision best left to trained medical practitioners, not law school graduates.

As successive Republican presidents have appointed right-wing ideologues to the court (although the Senate has summoned up the will to block ultra-right nominees like former Solicitor General Robert Bork, who fired Watergate special prosecutor Archibald Cox on President Nixon's orders after the president's Attorney General Elliot L. Richardson and his deputy, William D. Ruckelshaus, both refused to do so and resigned in protest over what came to be known as the "Saturday Night Massacre," and the unqualified, partisan George Bush crony, former White House counsel Harriet E. Miers, who has been directly implicated in the scandalous firing of eight U.S. attorneys who didn't demonstrate sufficient right-wing ardor), slightly less reactionaries like Justice Antonin Scalia who believes school districts should have the right to fire gay teachers even though the darling of the right, then Governor Reagan, denounced a California ballot initiative in the 1970s that would have driven out such teachers and his influence persuaded voters to kill the initiative, or Justice Clarence Thomas, who has declared his opposition to all forms of abortion and is notorious for falling asleep during post-lunch hearings, have somehow managed to overcome the exhaustion of the Democratic opposition and receive Senate confirmation of their appointments to the Supreme Court, it's only a matter of time before liberal justices retire or die, and their conservative replacements will at last muster the votes to overturn Roe vs. Wade.

What To Do About So-called "Strict Constructionist" Supreme Court Justices Who Legislate From the Bench

A national referendum once and for all will stop the creeping erosion of abortion rights and end the Supreme Court's consistent decisions that declare gun control legislation unconstitutional, citing the Second Amendment's alleged permission for every citizen to bear arms, even though gun control advocates insist that the amendment specifically limits gun ownership to militias, not private citizens who commit atrocities like the Columbine and Virginia Tech bloodbaths.

Unfortunately, the Second Amendment was purposely written in an ambiguous manner to allow legislators to reinterpret it differently and adapt it as social mores evolved during the following centuries of the Republic. In fact, most of the U.S. Constitution was left open to broad interpretation to accommodate this political and social evolution.

The entire text of the Second Amendment is only one sentence long: "A well regulated militia, being necessary to the security of a free state, the right of the people to keep and bear arms, shall not be infringed." It's not only ambiguous but ungrammatical—surprising since it was written by a scholar and Renaissance man, James Madison. Gun-owners have hijacked the Second Amendment's ambiguity and interpret it to mean that private citizens, not just militias who were needed to protect American revolutionaries against well-armed British invaders, have the right to arm themselves to the teeth.

While elected officials have sold their souls to the NRA in return for campaign contributions, even more egregiously silent on this moral issue and others have been church groups, especially the Evangelical right. In the Bible, Jesus said to turn the other cheek, not buy guns and shoot innocent people. Too many religions have kept their distance from other moral issues as well. Where is the clerical outrage on poverty, the lack of universal healthcare, its unequal distribution, and the inequitable distribution of wealth?

The New Testament's Book of Acts reveals that early Christians lived communally and shared their wealth. By that definition, Evangelicals and other conservative faiths aren't even Christian. Instead of following Jesus' other injunction to "judge ye not and ye shall not be judged" and "let those among you without sin cast the first stone," Christian fundamentalists have made a fetish of judging, i.e. condemning, alleged sinners who fail to follow their moral precepts. A good example of genuine Christianity is Mother Theresa, who denied herself, gave everything to the poor in India, lived with them on a daily basis at the same level of poverty, helping to feed the hungry and caring for the sick. Neither the Christian fundamentalists nor I come close to her self-sacrificing the example she set for the rest of us. I concede that I have been judgmental about many groups, including Evangelicals and politicians, but I'm not pretending to be a better individual than any of them. However, I am criticizing the hypocritical lives of those who pretend to be something they are not and judge others harshly.

Where is the churches' denunciation of fanatics who assassinate doctors at abortion clinics? Where does the Bible order its adherents to invade a non-threatening country, collude in the deaths of 20,000 Iraqis and the wounding of 100,000 more, while destroying the nation's infrastructure and failing to protect the lives of innocent civilians against fanatic religious radicals? These are not unjustifiable questions about Evangelicals' and other faiths' moral culpability for not only failing to condemn violence in all its various incarnations, but actively supporting it.

The hypocrisy of conservative politicians and their lack of compassion may be even more reprehensible than their religious coevals'. Republicans have blocked every attempt by Democrats to raise the obscenely low minimum of wage of $5.25 per hour and raise it to the still unlivable amount of $7.25 while in the last five to ten years, members of both parties have voted themselves wage increases averaging $50,000 *per annum*. Members of Congress should try living on five bucks an hour for a year and discover how impossible it is to survive on that amount. That would allow them to experience first-hand the quiet desperation, as Thoreau put it, that the working poor have had to endure.

This work may seem unfairly harsh on Republicans, but that's because until 2006, they had been in power for 12 years and blocked every effort to ameliorate the conditions of the poor and even the ever-dwindling numbers of the middle class as they find themselves sliding further and further down the socio-economic ladder. Adjusted for inflation, the middle class was far better off financially in the 1970s than it is today. For the poor, the decline in their standard of living has been even more severe and shameful.

If the Democrats remain in power, within four to six years they will demonstrate the same uncaring indifference as the Republicans have, which explains why Lord Acton's claim that power corrupts, absolute power corrupts absolutely continues to be quoted even though he made that comment almost a century ago. Although he was slightly exaggerating the similarities, Ralph Nader was close to the truth when he justified his establishment of the Green Party by insisting that there was no difference between the two major parties, or as novelist and essayist Gore Vidal put it, "There is only one party; it just has liberal and conservative wings." That is why the founding of a genuinely different third and/or fourth party is so critical.

The Hypocrisy and Ugliness of Personal Campaign Attacks

Besides eliminating or at least lessening the influence of special interests, we need to take the "personal" out of political debates, i.e. attacks on candidates' private lives which have no bearing on their ability to be effective legislators or chief executives. Hypocrisy often infuses these personal attacks. Perhaps the most outrageous incidence of hypocrisy came from former Republican Speaker of the House Newt Gingrich, who demanded President Clinton's impeachment because he lied under oath about his adulterous affair with Monica Lewinsky. Two years ago, *Vanity Fair* magazine "outed" Gingrich for carrying on an affair with his secretary while still married.

Gingrich's argument was similar and as ludicrous as Clinton's claim that he smoked but never inhaled marijuana. Only recently, as he considers a race for the presidency, has Gingrich finally admitted in public that he was just as guilty of adultery as President Clinton, and his only justification for his condemnation of Clinton's extra-marital behavior and not his own fling was that Gingrich never perjured himself by denying his affair ("I screwed but never lied"), which may be because he was never asked to testify before a grand jury about what goes on in his bedroom—and according to *Vanity Fair* in one incident on a desktop in his Congressional office.

The current fashion for *ad hominem* attacks against political opponents seems to be growing more risible and vicious by the day, often degenerating into self-parody, such as the time Barack Obama was denounced for his failure to pay 70 decades-old parking tickets or the spurious claim that he once was a Muslim because he attended a Muslim religious school or *madrassas* when he lived in Indonesia.

Obama has even been taken to task for sneaking cigarettes after promising his wife, in return for her support of his presidential bid, to give up nicotine. Another example of the viciousness of personal attacks was the ads paid for by Veterans for Swift Boat Truth—fellow Democrats (!) who claimed that Senator John Kerry was never wounded while he patrolled the waters of Vietnam even though Kerry to this day carries shrapnel in his body from attacks endured during his war-time patrols. Accurate but irrelevant to his qualifications to be president of the United States was the revelation that during a Vietnam War era protest, Kerry tore off and threw away the two Purple Heart medals he won for the same injuries which the Swift Boat partisans claimed he never sustained.

Some mudslinging is so petty it would be laughable if it were not so effective in trashing candidates' reputations and diminishing their electability. In his blog on the website *The First Post* in April 2007, left-wing commentator Alexander Cockburn quotes one of our least intellectually respected presidents, Calvin Coolidge, who said, "Any man who does not like dogs and not want them about does not deserve to be in the White House."

Extrapolating from Silent Cal's fatuous requirement to be Commander in Chief, Cockburn wrote, apparently tongue-out-of-cheek, "It looks like curtains for the Giuliani campaign," after the columnist revealed that Giuliani's third and current wife, Judi, "was once in the dog-killing business." Never mind that Judi's alleged pet atrocities occurred when she was 19 and married to her first husband, a salesman at a concern called U.S. Surgical. Judi was also an employee of the company, which sold veterinarian surgical staples, and among her duties was cutting open anesthetized dogs, whose wounds would then be closed up with surgical staples during sales-demonstrations for veterinarians.

The purpose of those promotional demonstrations is puzzling, because according to Patricia Feral, president of Friends of Animals in Connecticut, these canine guinea pigs often died during the procedure or had to be euthanized immediately after Judi wielded her machete on them because they couldn't recover from the surgery. Not a good marketing outcome. During the 1970s, 80s and 90s, Feral claimed that hundreds of dogs perished in this four-legged holocaust committed by Dr. Judi Mengele and fellow employees at U.S. Surgical. This was a cheap shot, and instead of concentrating on the unnecessary war initiated by Bush, which will eventually cause 4,000 American casualties, political pundits like Cockburn dredge up 20-year-old incidents which are irrelevant and of no value at this time. Justifiably, Rudy Giuliani's spokesman refused comment on his wife's murderous past, which was first reported on the *New York Post's* website.

Campaigns should return to the past custom of civility. They should stress the positive over the negative, debating the important issues and proposing legislation that will improve the welfare of the American people.

There is no need for negative attacks against opponents, irrelevant mud-slinging and uncovering 40-year-old missteps like Albert Gore smoking marijuana in college and Barack Obama using both marijuana and cocaine during the typical reckless years of youthful indulgence.

As George Bush's clever tautology excusing transgressions in his 20s during the 2000 presidential campaign had it, "When I was young and irresponsible, I was young and irresponsible," failing to reveal that his youthful actions were more than just irresponsible and involved two driving under the influence convictions that endangered the lives of three passengers, including family members, while he sat behind the wheel intoxicated. As the classic bumper stick notes, "Nobody died when Clinton lied," which cannot be said about the presidential prevarications that induced members of Congress, much to their later regret and embarrassment, to support Bush's invasion of Iraq. Candidates should behave like civilized adults, focusing on the positive rather than the negative.

To recap, here are 10 easy-to-follow recommendations that should be heeded by all elected officials:

1. Remind Congress and the White House that they are honored to serve the American people they represent. Government service is not a decades-long career or a sinecure to make a killing from. The exigencies of their jobs demand sacrifice and compromise in their personal lives, including spending less time with their families and more time on the floor of the Senate and the House of Representatives. Too many politicians flee Washington on early Thursday morning to return to their home districts and don't return until Monday afternoon!

2. Be honest, have integrity, avoid hypocrisy, be yourself and stop pretending to espouse principles you personally don't believe in but promote for the sake of political expediency and reelection.

3. Remember: you are serving the people, not your party which leads us to:

4. Be willing to cross party lines and support legislation that benefits the American people rather than lemming-like subservience to your party's leaders and ideologues.

5. Remain open-minded, achieve the goals of the American people. Don't have a narrow-minded attitude. Reject irrelevant ideology that only pleases minority but powerful special interests.

6. Be independent of outside influences. Don't allow yourself to be bought by lobbyists so you can think and move freely.

7. Try to make deals with colleagues from across the aisle and move legislation along instead of blocking it for partisan motives.

8. Stop slinging mud at opponents and focus on issues, not personalities. During close elections especially, avoid the temptation to dig up ancient dirt on your opponents, no matter how fierce the race turns out to be. Let the people elect or reelect you based on your achievements and legislative track record rather than just presenting yourself as the less objectionable alternative to your opponent.

9. Focus on the main issues that will benefit the American people, like healthcare, education, poverty, crime reduction and national security. Collateral issues like abortion and gay rights only reflect the preoccupations of unrepresentative special interests and do not promote the welfare of the general public.

10. Treat the U.S. Treasury like your personal family bank account. Spend tax revenues wisely and effectively for the benefit of taxpayers who contribute to the Treasury.

Political reform is not a one-way street, and American voters also have responsibilities already described in the text and summarized here:

1. Be independent in your decisions. Don't let special interest groups like the NRA, the Evangelical right and corporate powerhouses influence your vote. Ignore the will of the political base of both parties and vote your conscience.

2. Be a good citizen and research the main issues facing America today that will help your country, your family and yourself.

3. Be an American first and a Democrat or Republican second. Vote as an American, not as a partisan.

4. Try to encourage independent or third party candidates even if they have less media exposure due to lack of funding by special interest groups.

5. Limit incumbents to two terms in the Senate (12 years) and Congressmen to four terms (eight years). Elect new people with fresh ideas. Long-time incumbents make the political process stagnant and vulnerable to corruption. They tend to block legislation opposed by their financial benefactors, be they corporate interests, the radical religious right or the leaders of their own parties. There is no justification for spending decades in Congress because representing the people is not a career, it's a public service, like serving on the board of a philanthropical organization. Congressmen who stay in office more than a quarter of a century have irrelevant ideas that do not reflect the concerns of the current generation.

6. The present two-party system has miserably failed and thwarted the wishes of the American people. Make donations to third-party candidates; don't give up on them quickly because of poor showings in early polls, which is what typically dooms independent candidates' electoral bids. Be patient, stay the course, and give third-party hopefuls the time to prove themselves during debates and stump speeches which will eventually allow them to rise in the polls.

7. Try to recruit good candidates and induce them to join a third party.

8. Get involved in political activities. Attend political meetings so you can understand the issues. Al Gore's 2000 defeat by a tiny margin of electoral (not popular) vote proved the importance of each and every vote. Your vote is valuable. Be a good citizen and

go the polls on every election day, including primaries and mid-term elections.

9. Do not contribute financially to the major parties who are backed by special interests. Encourage friends and family to contribute to third-party candidates or to an election commission that will distribute funds equally rather than matching the enormous amount of funds that only major party candidates can raise. Matching campaign funds are a self-perpetuating process that keeps the same mediocrities in office year after year. Contributions to independents or to an electoral commission can be as little as $5 and still make a difference in a candidate's viability. Five to ten dollars per person deducted from income taxes will create a potent war chest of $1.5 billion every year and a whopping $5.2 billion every four years, based on an American population of 300 million. This will not be a flat tax but a graduated one. There can be three tax brackets: based on income, the top 20 percent of the population will be required to contribute $10 per person, the middle income bracket will pay $5, and the poorest segment will pay nothing. One fourth of the amount raised by this electoral tax will go to presidential candidates evenly, and the remaining three quarters will go to those running for the Senate and House. These funds should be paid in three increments: ten months, six months and three months prior to the general election, so that candidates who remain viable in the polls as the campaign progresses will receive more and more funds because of the dwindling number of contenders. Their increased funding will reflect the choice of the American people as they reject candidates during the primary season. Only candidates who refuse outside funding should be eligible for this windfall. Campaigners who do accept non-government financial contributions can be "shamed" into rejecting funds offered by special interests with the help of the media, which will publish the amount and source of outside donations. A tally of outside financial aid should be revealed every three months, so the public will know who has already been

bought by special interests and not vote for them. Hillary Clinton is a good example of someone who has been embarrassed into returning contributions to her campaign from an Islamic anti-Israel organization.

10. And finally, vote for candidates who demonstrate genuine, not expedient, integrity and honesty and whose agenda is to improve the lives of their constituents. Forgive and forget sins committed 20 or 30 years ago since most people misbehaved during their youth and reform themselves upon maturity. President Bush gave up drinking alcohol at the age of 40 after his wife threatened to leave him. Family matters and private life should not be dredged up.

Establishing third and fourth parties is admittedly a long shot, and all similar attempts have failed in the past. Indeed, the last successful third party, the Republican, was inaugurated way back in 1856. Four years later, the new party captured the presidency, and with a few exceptions, retained control of the presidency and both houses of Congress until Democrat Woodrow Wilson recaptured the presidency in 1912.

In the past 15 years, during each presidential election, a third party arrives on the scene then quickly vanishes. Third party candidates seem to be as ephemeral as a lit candle. There are many reasons for the successive failures of third parties gaining a permanent foothold among the electorate. First, the public was not effectively educated (read indoctrinated) about the necessity of a third party. In 1992, Ross Perot's Reform Party managed to hold the public's attention for two to four years, then its influence waned and the American people, notorious for their short attention span, lost interest in Perot and the principles of his party. Perot was partially to blame for the Reform Party's demise because he failed to generate and sustain media interest. His "15 minutes of fame" didn't last longer than one election cycle.

Second, many third party candidates are defectors from one of the main parties, and if they can't even win the nomination with all the assistance they derive from their majority party affiliation, how can they possibly hope to win as a third party candidate with that party's lesser resources and clout? Paleolithic conservatives like Pat Buchanan failed to win the presidential Republican party nomination, defected to Perot's party and garnered votes in the low single-figures. Donald Trump also unsuccessfully put himself forward as a Reform Party candidate, but his campaign was never taken seriously and was considered by many a publicity stunt by a man who never met a camera lens he didn't love. (Note his continuing grudge match with TV personality Rosie O'Donnell over non-existent issues. At least it gets his name in print and his face on TV.)

The eccentric Jesse Ventura, a former pro-wrestler and the unlikely governor of Minnesota, also failed miserably in his third party bid for the presidency. Other third party hopefuls never manage to gain traction because they get pigeon-holed as single-issue candidates and do not communicate effectively the other planks in their party's platforms.

In 2000 and 2004, Green Party presidential candidate Ralph Nader became identified with only one issue—the environment—while in fact his party promoted many other issues but didn't manage to lodge them in the national consciousness. It takes time—often decades—for a third party to establish itself as a viable political organization, but the more voters understand the necessity of an alternative party to unblock Congressional gridlock and dilute the power of well-heeled special interests, the faster a third party will become a major and not a fringe player.

The party platform should resemble diners at a buffet: adopt the best issues of both major parties and discard the bad. Keeping an open mind, unlike the ossified members of the Democratic and Republican parties, the third party will eventually become a mainstream contender, uncorrupted by corporate powerbrokers. They will be a party *of* the people and *for* the people as our Founding Fathers intended.

Someone who has already failed on the Republican or Democratic ticket can't expect to win as a third party candidate. A third party needs fresh faces with new ideas and famous, charismatic personnel, not failed retreads from the major parties. A notable exception to this phenomenon was the successful candidacy of Senator Joe Lieberman of Connecticut, who didn't win renomination as a Democrat because of his reactionary ideology, most notably his puzzling support of the war in Iraq as well as his cranky denunciations of minor issues like TV and film violence, but ran as an independent and won. However, reflecting the impotence of independents and third party candidates, as soon as Lieberman was reelected to the Senate, he retreated to the safe (and more powerful) refuge of the Democratic party.

But history is not destiny. If a third party doesn't succeed in getting on the ballot, there is another way to end the gridlock, corruption and control by special interests that currently plague our representatives in the nation's capital. And that is simply to make an end run around Congress and cut them out of the equation. The chronic problems that are never solved by legislators can be overcome by the creation of a national referendum which would be held every 25 to 50 years.

Abortion, gay rights, gun control, and saving Social Security from insolvency when the baby boom generation turns 65, are all issues that in the past 30 years come up at every election—presidential, congressional and gubernatorial. Politicians intensely debate these problems and make promises to fix them during the campaign season, but as soon as they get elected or reelected to office they suffer collective amnesia and the issues are never heard from again.

Remember when candidate Bush promised to balance the budget when he ran for president in 2000 and instead, once he got into office, cut taxes and spent billions waging the war in Iraq, which caused the federal budget, once balanced by President Clinton so effectively that he generated a surplus, to run up huge deficits that our luckless grandchildren will be burdened with for decades to come? It's comparable to private citizens passing on massive credit card debt to their kids and grandkids after they die.

It may seem difficult if not next to impossible to get Congress to put a national referendum on the ballot every 25 to 50 years, especially if the referendum contains such loathed provisions as term limits and the end of corporate funding of political campaigns. Incumbents are unlikely to vote themselves out of office, but there is a way to overcome Congressional resistance to a referendum, and it has to do with the crucial establishment of a third party.

With the support and encouragement of this party, voters will chuck the current majority party candidates out of office, and the third party, with help from defectors from the major parties (much as a handful of Republican defectors today have crossed the aisle and sided with Democrats on withdrawing from Iraq), will place the referendum on the ballot. Voters can help too. They should put the incumbents who resist the referendum on notice that they will not be returned to office in the next election unless they agree to a referendum. Successful third party candidates will initiate the referendum, and incumbents who want to stay in power will be compelled to back them.

Perhaps most effectively of all, a national referendum will once and for all tackle the intractable problem of gun ownership and the human havoc it causes. The disturbed gunman who killed 32 students at Virginia Tech in April 2007 legally bought both the handguns he used in his rampage at gun shops. He simply lied on the application form that asked if he had ever been institutionalized for mental health reasons, which he had.

The gun lobby cites such easily faked answers as proof that gun control doesn't work and that criminals will ignore the law while law-abiding citizens disarm themselves and become defenseless against armed perpetrators. A majority of Americans want handguns now owned by private citizens banned outright. Even typically conservative law enforcement officers want guns outlawed because so many of their co-workers have been killed by weapons purchased legally. The police are tired of being target practice for demented shooters. The NRA, which has enormous political influence because of its huge campaign war chest, has successfully deflected all legislative attempts to limit or eliminate private gun ownership for decades.

A national referendum can make an end-run around the NRA by banning the possession of handguns. Although it seems inexplicable that hunters derive gratification from killing magnificent and defenseless game animals. (How can a civilized human being shoot a graceful deer or majestic elk? It's like blowing away a Great Dane or Mastiff.) But a referendum will provide a compromise with die-hard hunters that will also keep dangerous rifles out of the hands of madmen by requiring hunters to check their weapons in a public storage facility, where they will only be permitted to retrieve them on hunting day. The Beverly Hills Gun Club, which boasts member such as Sylvester Stallone and Sharon Stone, already provides a facility where hunters can stash their rifles, but the practice currently is on a voluntary basis. A national referendum would make it mandatory.

Grim Polls

Successive surveys prove the urgent need to end gridlock in Washington and the legislative and executive branches' unresponsiveness to the will of the American people.

A May 2007 poll conducted by the Associated Press indicated that only 25 percent of Americans approved of the direction in which the nation is headed, the lowest level since AP started gauging citizens' dissatisfaction with the U.S. government in 2003, the year Bush's adventurism in Iraq began.

In fact, the majority of the poll's 1,000 respondents attributed their displeasure with the state of the state to the war. Only nine percent of those polled blamed the economy, which was enjoying an historically low level of 2.3 per cent annual inflation a month before the May 2007 AP poll, and an unemployment rate of 4.5 percent in April 2007, also historically low. Eight percent of respondents criticized the loss of moral values—a tiny percentage of moral outrage which again proves how out of touch the Christian right is with the concerns of mainstream Americans. And surprisingly only five percent faulted gasoline prices despite the fact that fuel costs were at an all-time high in early May 2007 at $3.07 per gallon of regular unleaded—still a pittance compared to astronomical pump prices in oil-deprived Europe, where the U.K. in April 2007 was charging $7.10 per gallon. No wonder horses are so popular in England.

Other polls conducted about the same time as the AP survey demonstrated that Republican presidential candidates are paying the highest price for their lame-duck leader's policies. These polls revealed that the majority of Americans prefer a Democrat occupy the White House after the 2008 election—without naming which Democratic, probably reflecting the neck-and-neck race between Hillary Clinton and Barack Obama. There was good news from these surveys for at least one Republican presidential hopeful, however. Rudy Giuliani in May 2007 was holding his own against Clinton and Obama. Giuliani's stellar ranking compared to his trailing Republican opponents' may be due to his liberal political platform, which isn't that much different from the planks of the leading Democratic contenders.

CHAPTER FOUR
Saving American Foreign Policy

All the current bills to end the war in Iraq will never become law because the Democrats don't have the votes to override President Bush's inevitable veto and not enough Republicans are willing to defect to the Democrats' position on ending the war. The gravity and urgency of this issue cannot be overemphasized. An April 2007 poll reported that 64 percent of the American people call the war "a mistake." What a difference time and four years of carnage make.

On May 2, 2003, a little over a month after U.S. and British troops invaded Iraq from Kuwait and toppled Saddam Hussein, the President gave a speech on the deck of the U.S.S. Abraham Lincoln aircraft carrier docked at San Diego, standing in front of an enormous banner with a slo-gan that would turn out to be tragically ironic: "Mission Accomplished." At the time, "only" 139 American soldiers had lost their lives in the con-flict and two-thirds of the American public approved of the President's prosecution of the war.

By the fourth-year anniversary of that speech, the same day the Presi-dent vetoed a House-Senate funding bill that also called for the withdrawal of American troops from Iraq, 3,213 servicemen and women had perished, and only one-third of the people gave Bush a positive job approval rating.

Probably this group consists largely of Republicans, including the Evangel-ical right, who blindly support the war.

If that same 64 percent of disenchanted voters were reflected in the composition of the Senate membership, anti-war legislators would have enough votes to end Republican filibusters and need only three more votes to override a presidential veto.

But until the number of Senators who oppose the war catches up to the percentage of American voters who agree with these doves, there is another way around filibustering hawks. With as little as 10 percent representation in both houses, a minority third or fourth party could join forces with either of the major parties and pass any legislation currently blocked by fil-ibuster and veto.

Prior to the creation of a third party, which may take years and we don't have time to let the death toll continue in Iraq for that long, voters, by responding to national polls, can put Republican proponents of con-tinuing the Iraq war on notice that if they don't cross the aisle and join forces with anti-war Democrats, the Republican hawks will be turned out of office in the next election.

One of the many benefits of term limits discussed in Chapter One have already proved themselves brilliantly in the case of power-hungry presi-dents who might be tempted to run for a third term like FDR, who won four. The war in Iraq will never end until President Bush leaves office after his second term. The leading presidential contenders in the 2008 election have all promised in their political platforms to stop the war ASAP.

Senator Barack Obama has said he will complete withdrawal of our troops within a year of his election, and Senator Hillary Clinton plans to end American involvement within two. Sadly, if the current casualty rates of American troops continue while we wait for President Bush's departure, another 1,000 to 2,000 men and women in uniform will die during that time.

That's a profoundly depressing tragedy that can't be overcome until 2008 at the earliest. In the meantime, young people with their whole lives ahead of them will return from Iraq broken in mind or body. An estimated

10 percent of Iraqi war veterans suffer from post traumatic stress disorder, an intractable psychological problem almost impossible to treat.

Post-Mortem on Iraq

The conflict in Iraq may enjoy the dubious distinction of being the dumbest war in the history of the Republic, even topping the lunacy of our earlier attempt to stop a similar civil war and defeat an undefeatable guerilla force in Vietnam. Armchair psychologists have speculated that President Bush decided to invade Iraq because Saddam Hussein had allegedly put a hit out on his father during a visit to Kuwait by the elder Bush in 1993.

The problem with this pop Freudian theory is that Bush *fils* has very little love for Bush *père*, so George Jr. would be unlikely to launch a massive vendetta against a man (Hussein) who tried to kill another man (George Sr.) he doesn't particularly care for. The ill will between our 41st and 43rd president has been documented with relish by the more gossipy elements of the media.

Regardless of whatever subterranean reasons motivated our inscrutable Commander in Chief to oust Hussein, his decision was aided and abetted by either fabricated or unsubstantiated intelligence provided by an incompetent CIA and NSA (National Security Agency) that Iraq not only possessed weapons of mass destruction, an allegation which did enjoy some credibility because Hussein had used such weapons against his Kurdish and Shiite citizens during uprisings in 1981, and the even more inflammatory claim that Hussein had colluded with Al Qaeda in the 9/11 attacks.

The opportunistic long-time Iraqi exile and convicted felon Ahmed Chalabi, the darling of the Defense Department, misled the President by predicting that American forces, like the GIs who marched into Paris in 1944, would be treated like liberators and greeted with flowers and chocolates by the oppressed Shiite majority. Innocently or purposely, the so-called neocon experts who orchestrated the invasion disastrously miscalculated the real aftermath of the Iraq incursion.

By now, a majority of Americans, but unfortunately still not a majority of Republican legislators (because they represent the will of their party's masters, not the will of the people) believe that the war was a mistake.

However, the number of Republicans who still support the policy of their chief in the White House seems to be decreasing with almost daily media reports of yet more defections by members of the President's own party.

A Sinking Ship of War

Like rats deserting a sinking Presidency, even some of the President's men—most surprisingly his Secretary of Defense, Robert M. Gates—have crossed over to the Democratic side, which supports timetables for the withdrawal of troops in Iraq—anathema to what novelist Gore Vidal has called the "Cheney-Bush *Junta*."

According to a report in the May 6, 2007, edition of the *Los Angeles Times*, during a visit to the Middle East, Gates told members of the Iraqi government and later a U.S. press conference that he agreed with Democrats' insistence on pulling our troops out of Iraq. Gates even wants that withdrawal to take place sooner than some dovish Democrats. While most Democrats call for beginning withdrawal by October 1, 2007, a former senior Defense official claims Gates is even more impatient about waiting to determine if the troop surge is working. "[Gates] wants to see some results by summer, and if he doesn't see those results, he seems willing to throw the towel in," the former official said. Even the Iraq Study Group, which Gates was a member of until Bush appointed him Secretary of Defense, was willing to give the President until early 2008 to initiate troop withdrawal.

Supporters of Bush's position have slammed Gates for undercutting his Commander in Chief. "You shortchange the President's plan if you rush to judge its [the surge's] effects prematurely. De facto you are undermining the strategy," a former member of the Defense Department said.

Several prominent Congressional Republicans have also seen the light as prospects for their reelection in 2008 grow dimmer. Liberal Republican Senator Susan Collins of Maine, who voted against the Democratic Iraq funding bill Bush vetoed in May 2007, has had a change of heart and begun work on legislation that would force the Iraqi government to meet certain goals if it wants continued U.S. funding. Collins' about face may have come too late. She is trailing her Democratic rival in the polls.

Rep. Charles Boustany, Jr., a Republican from Louisiana, also opposed the Democratic funding bill but has now become another defector from the White House position and says, "We have to be engaged developing our own proposals and not just going along with what the executive branch is doing."

The influential former chairman of the Senate Armed Services Committee, Republican Senator John W. Warner of Virginia, was one of the few members of Bush's party to oppose his sending an additional 21,500 troops to pacify Baghdad and Al Anbar Province in January 2007.

Since then, he has moved even further away from the President's position. Warner said in May 2007 that he was working on a compromise bill that would appeal to both parties and attract the magic number of 70 votes—enough to override the inevitable veto by the President of any legislation that sets benchmarks and timetables for withdrawal. "I'm optimistic something can be worked out," Warner said.

Bush stalwarts, like South Carolina Republican Senator Lindsey Graham, are still playing the disloyalty card and accusing doves of undercutting our troops in Iraq, an argument that by 2007 had lost much of its emotional punch. " ... when you set timelines, deadlines and denying funding, you're basically empowering the enemy to make sure you fail," Graham said.

As the number of Iraqis tortured and killed by both Shiite death squads and Sunni insurgents increases despite the troop buildup at the beginning of 2007, critics of the war say too late, we've already failed.

Bush Gives In—or a Snowball's Chance in Hell?

In April 2007, President Bush vetoed a bill providing additional funds for the war in Iraq, in part because the legislation tied continued funding to "benchmarks"—milestones and timetables that require the Iraqi government to show progress on sharing oil wealth among Shiites, Sunnis and Kurds, disarm sectarian militias and further reduce violence between Sunnis and Shiites, among other benchmarks.

After a mob of moderate Senators from both parties descended on the White House in May 2007 to share their dissatisfaction with Bush's management of the war and another gang of 11 Republican Congressmen warned him that the conflict was undermining public support for their party, Bush dumbfounded his audience at a Pentagon press conference on May 10, 2007, by appearing to do an about—face and agree to benchmarks. "One message I have heard from people from both parties is that the idea of benchmarks makes sense. And I agree," Bush said at the Pentagon briefing.

No, he doesn't.

It seemed as though Bush had finally come around to the side of his critics, but then he immediately equivocated by adding that he would not accept any new funding bill that included benchmarks, in effect, nullifying the promise he had just made at the Pentagon to allow such provisions.

Bush's implicit threat to veto yet again any bill tying troop funding to benchmarks didn't deter a bipartisan coalition of Senators from proposing just such a bill. After Bush's appearance at the Pentagon, allies from both sides of the aisle, Republican Senator Lamar Alexander of Tennessee and Democratic Senator Ken Salazar of Colorado, promised to introduce legislation that would cut funding for American troops if the Iraqi government didn't reach certain milestones. But not only Republican politicians wary of losing reelection by hitching their wagon to Bush's imploding star have deserted the President. Two Army generals, including one active duty officer—the No. 2 man in Iraq, have publicly criticized the President's handling of the war.

In May 2007, retired Major General John Batiste, the former commander of the First Infantry Division in Iraq, appeared in a TV commercial that aired in Republican Congressional districts as part of a $500,000 effort funded by VoteVets.org. Batiste told TV audiences, "Mr. President, you did not listen. You continue to pursue a failed strategy that is breaking our great Army and Marine Corps. I left the Army [three years ago] in protest in order to speak out. Mr. President, you have placed our nation in peril. Our only hope is that Congress will act now to protect our fighting men and women." Other retired officers, including 2004 Democratic presidential contender, former General Wesley K. Clark, have also criticized Bush, but Batiste's comments were notable for their severity.

Emily Lawrimore, an official in the White House's Office of Communications, responding to Batiste's charge that Bush "did not listen," claimed that the President routinely conferred with senior officers, including the Joint Chiefs of Staff, as well as with General David H. Petraeus, the leader of American troops in Iraq.

Bush apparently has not conferred with the No. 2 man in Iraq, Army Major General Benjamin R. Mixon, the commander of U.S. forces in the northern region of that country. Bush deployed an additional 21,500 military personnel in January 2007 to pacify Baghdad and Al Anbar province. In a news teleconference at the Pentagon on May 11, 2007, Batiste, speaking from Iraq, noted that the surge had had just the opposite of its intended effect. "The level of violence [in Baghdad] began to increase before the surge. It has increased during the surge."

The *New York Times* said it was rare for an officer of Mixon's rank to criticize his Commander in Chief, and the *Times* categorized as "withering" the general's denunciation of the Iraqi government as hamstrung by bureaucracy and compromised by corruption and sectarian discord, which has made the government unable to assist U.S. forces in pacifying Iraq.

Retired Army Maj. Gen. William L. Nash offered a theory for the atypical harshness of Mixon's comments. Former Secretary of Defense Donald H. Rumsfeld, Nash said, "intensely pressured" field officers to refrain from criticizing the President, even in private. Nash attributed this new frankness to the current Defense Secretary, Robert M. Gates. Nash said, "I suspect the new Defense Secretary has told general officers to speak their minds." As already noted, Gates himself has done just that—calling for a pullout from Iraq earlier than even some Democratic doves have demanded.

Maybe it was Gates' encouragement that led yet another officer in the field, Lt. Col. Paul Yingling, deputy commander of the 3rd Armored Cavalry Regiment, in a May 2007 article in the *Armed Forces Journal*, to blast the top brass in Iraq for "botching the war and misleading the American public and Congress."

History's Ignoramuses

There was no threat posed by Hussein against the U.S., no threat of terrorists in Iraq who might attempt a copycat massacre like 9/11. The late Harvard philosopher Georges Santayana said that those who do not learn the mistakes of the past are condemned to repeat them, and as the professor has been proven correct many times since then, the U.S. did not heed earlier political and military blunders.

History has taught us that fanatic terrorists do not flourish in totalitarian regimes like Saddam's or Gamal Abdul Nasser's in Egypt in the 1950s and 60s. As *The Opium Wars: The Addiction of One Empire and the Corruption of Another*, pointed out in 2002, after the Chinese had spent centuries unsuccessfully battling opium addiction, when the totalitarian Chairman Mao Tse-Teung came to power in 1949, he wiped out the drug's use within a generation simply by executing all opium dealers and addicts. Today, opium manufacture in China is miniscule and used for medicinal purposes and research only. Except for one assassination attempt by bumbling military officers, no one dared oppose Hitler during his so-called "thousand year Reich," which lasted only 12.

Disdainful of national aspirations, the Soviet Union also suppressed revolts by its Eastern European satellites for more than four decades because it didn't have to answer to a dovish opposition among its *nomenklatura*. Dictators are often ruthless sociopaths who run their countries as police states and don't have to answer to such niceties as our Bill of Rights or English Common Law.

Western democracies do not have the luxury of disregarding civil liberties that allows dictators to liquidate terrorists and other criminals without due process—although the *habeas corpus* abuses at Guantanamo Bay and Abu Ghraib suggest that the current administration—with such "no-brainer" comments approving the use of water board torture by Vice President Dick Cheney—does not worship at the same legal altar as the ACLU.

Al Qaeda never gained a foothold in Iraq because Hussein followed the German sociologist Max Weber's cynical assertion in his 1904 classic *The Protestant Ethic* that what defines a sovereign state—both democratic and repressive—is its monopoly on violence. Al Qaeda represented competition for Hussein's monopoly, and he suppressed it. This fact was known but conveniently ignored even before the U.S. began its Iraqi adventure in March 2003.

The second blunder the U.S. made (mistake No. 1 being the invasion itself) was the dismissal of the entire Iraqi army and police force because they were members of Hussein's Baath party. At the time, the blizzard of pink slips was blamed on L. Paul Bremer III, the head of the U.S.-led occupation government of Iraq from 2003 to 2004. But Bremer later testified before Congress that he was acting on orders from then Secretary of Defense Donald H. Rumsfeld.

The bulk of the army and police were not culpable or necessarily loyal to Hussein. They were afraid of the dictator, who made membership in the Baath party a condition of their employment. They had the additional incentive of receiving much higher pay than the average Iraqi civilian. If Rumsfeld had not dismissed the two services and instead had paid them as well as Hussein, they would have preserved order and stability and prevented internecine warfare just as they had done under the former dictator's regime.

The third mistake was that the U.S. military should have left one year after the 2003 invasion because Hussein had been captured, his two psychopathic sons killed in a shootout with American forces and most of the top Baath party membership was in prison. On May 1, 2007, Congress sent the President a spending bill ordering U.S. withdrawal from Iraq within a year, and as threatened, the President vetoed it.

Congress should respond by submitting another bill to Bush offering to finance the war for one more year, during which time the President will be able to prove whether or not the 21,500 troop surge which began in January 2007 has successfully pacified Iraq, and the Iraqi government will be able to prove that it can keep the country stable without the assistance of American troops.

In a June 2007 poll by the Washington-based think tank/website, World Public Opinion.org, 70 percent of Iraqis wanted the Americans out of their country, and 60 percent said they approved the killing of American military personnel. Gratitude. Or as Dorothy Parker apocryphally said, "No good deed goes unpunished."

World Public Opinion think tank speculated that Iraqi citizens' murderous resentment of the U.S. troop presence derives from the widely-held belief that the Bush administration plans to maintain permanent military bases in Iraq. With an ever-increasing chorus of Congressional members calling for withdrawal from Iraq, the Iraqi perception that Bush wants an open-ended commitment to remaining in their country may seem paranoid, but as Henry Kissinger conceded, "Even paranoid people have enemies."

And not-so-paranoid Iraqis can justify their fears by pointing to the President himself, who fueled their suspicions when Presidential spokesmen Tony Snow in June 2008 quotes his boss as being "intrigued" by the idea of applying the "Korean model" to Iraq. The Korean model refers to the fact that since 1954, when an armistice was signed ending hostilities between North Korea and the U.S., American troops have remained stationed in South Korea.

Although only a month earlier, Defense Secretary Robert M. Gates was sounding positively dovish when he called for an early troop draw down, Gates told the *New York Times* a day after Snow's statement that he supported the President's Korean analogy of keeping a long-term American garrison in Iraq instead of imitating the Vietnam model "where we just left lock, stock and barrel."

Bush's rejection of a timetable for withdrawal in favor of a permanent presence in Iraq seems to be moving in the opposite direction of American public opinion, some active duty U.S. military brass and an ever-expanding number of Congressional defectors from his own party. His long-time promise to "stay the course" has now been more specifically defined as "staying the course *indefinitely.*"

During the proposed one-year grace period Congress allows the President to prove the effectiveness of the troop surge, the U.S. should dramatically increase training of the Iraqi army and police to suppress both Sunni insurgents and Shiite death squads. By giving the President and Iraq 12 months to get their acts together, Bush will no longer be able to use the excuse that Congress wants to abandon U.S. troops by abruptly cutting off their funding—something Congress has never threatened to do.

One year is plenty of time for Bush to demonstrate the efficacy of the surge and plan a U.S. withdrawal. Bush's continued bull-headed insistence on "staying the course," a grotesque euphemism for allowing the carnage to continue indefinitely or at least until he leaves the Oval Office, must be thwarted by decisive action by our legislators. Sadly, even this one-year allowance means at least another 1,000 American servicemen and women at current casualty rates will needlessly be sacrificed and billions of dollars wasted. Regardless of whatever timetable for withdrawal is eventually accepted by the President, the end will come like South Vietnam's collapse in 1975—withdrawal without victory.

Let's hope that unlike Saigon in 1975, the U.S. will be better prepared and there will be no iconic imagery like the shameful sight of our desperate South Vietnamese allies climbing single file up the ladder of a lone helicopter evacuating refugees on the roof of the American embassy.

Beyond Iraq

Unlike our Iraqi policy, I am an enthusiastic supporter of the war in Afghanistan. My only regret is that then President Clinton didn't invade the nation which harbored Al Qaeda in 1998 after the terrorist group bombed two U.S. embassies in Africa. In 1998, Clinton should have imitated Bush's actions in 2001–2002 by bombarding Afghanistan. Unfortunately, with the current President's typical short attention span, within a year of the Afghani invasion, he transitioned from offensive to defensive mode in that country shortly before he overextended the capability of U.S. troops by starting another war in Iraq.

Bush's defensive repositioning in Afghanistan allowed Al Qaeda and its Taliban allies to mount offensive actions against American forces stationed on the Afghan/Pakistan border. Both radical Islamic groups began to regroup and flourish, while planning further attacks against the United States and executing attacks against our European allies in Spain and the United Kingdom. In a 2002 report in the on-line edition of *USA Today*, it quoted U.S. officials who claimed that Osama bin Laden in an audiotape "implied" that his operatives should attack 60 (!) countries.

U.S. troops should have maintained their offensive posture in Afghanistan for another one to two years in order to finish the job in that country by bombarding the Tora Bora mountains first, then advancing on both sides of the border between Afghanistan and Pakistan. The majority of terrorists in Afghanistan would have been liquidated by now if that policy had been pursued. The U.S. government also should have given Afghanistan an ultimatum that if it continued to harbor and collaborate with Al Qaeda, aerial bombardment would resume in the future.

But President Bush was afraid that such threats and attacks would have alienated America's equivocal ally, Pakistani President Pervez Musharraf. The American President considers his counterpart in Pakistan a friend of our country simply because he snatches one or two terrorists every three to six months and hands them over to us.

The U.S. is paying dearly for this less than diligent service. A May 20, 2007, front-page report in the *New York Times* revealed that the U.S. is giving the Pakistani dictator $1 to $10 billion per year to patrol the Afghan/Pakistan border, even though Musharraf in 2006 slashed the number of troops he sent to the region. To date, the U.S. has paid Pakistan many billions for "services not rendered."—the tab for this American largesse, according to the *Times*, "buried in public budget numbers." The Pentagon admitted that Musharraf is paid $80 million per month.

Gordon Johndroe, a spokesman for Stephen J. Hadley, the Whites House's national security adviser, justified the cost of this dubious military assistance: "Pakistan's cooperation is very important in the global war on terror and for our operations in Afghanistan. Our investments in that partnership have paid off over time, from increased information sharing to kills and captures of key terrorists operatives. There is more work to be done, the Pakistanis know that, and we are engaged with the Musharraf government to ramp up the fight."

Meanwhile, Al Qaeda and the Taliban are multiplying and regrouping in Pakistan at a faster rate than those captured by Musharraf. For every one or two terrorists apprehended, 100 take their place. At the same time, they have been exporting their ideology and activities by forming branches all over Europe, the Middle East and even in America. Rather than ending the terrorist threat by invading Iraq, the U.S. turned that country into a breeding ground and training camp for new members—Sunni insurgents—to attack American troops.

Because of this metastasis of terrorism, I fear another 9/11-style assault on America in the near future. Al Qaeda is coordinating this attack from the safety of its refuge on the Afghan/Pakistani border. When the almost inevitable repeat of 9/11 occurs, whether or not President Bush is still in office, he will be blamed for 9/11 redux just as President Clinton was lambasted for not dealing with Osama bin Laden before the Al Qaeda leader was able to mastermind the World Trade Center tragedy.

Bush will dredge up the same excuses for failing to preempt 9/11 II as Clinton did after two American embassies in Africa were bombed. Also like Clinton, Bush will insist he did everything possible—except succeed. Immediately, Bush must begin annihilating the terrorist pockets, including their training camps, on the Pakistani side of the border and publicize the threat that if the terrorist return to their activities, American forces will return and again attack by air, land and sea. Our troops must eventually and sooner rather than later exit Afghanistan and spare the families of American soldiers the agony of a war that has dragged on for six disgraceful years.

The Mess in the Middle East

I was born in Egypt in 1941 and lived there for the next 28 years. Although I am an Orthodox Coptic Christian by birth, I attended public schools in my native land and learned about Islamic religion and culture. Along with my fellow Muslim students, I studied the Koran more as Arabic literature (which was a curriculum requirement) than as a theological text. My Muslim peers in our neighborhood enrolled in the same schools, and we worked together after graduating from college. I dare to say I am thoroughly knowledgeable about Arabic, Muslim and Middle Eastern culture in general.

From grade school through medical school, the student body was then approximately 20 to 25 percent Christian and 75 to 80 percent Muslim. So I believe I can say with no immodesty that I understand the mindset and culture of Muslims, especially the manner in which they react to perceived insults against their religion like the cartoons that appeared first in Denmark and then in other European countries lampooning the prophet Mohammed.

In 1969, I emigrated to England, where I remained in contact for the next two to three years with many fellow expatriate Middle Easterners with whom I became friends. Because of my many Muslim and Middle Eastern Christian associates, I know how they think and in particular what things really enrage them. My background makes me more informed than the average U.S.-born citizen about Middle Easterners because I lived with them in both Egypt and Europe.

In 1971 I moved again, to the United States and have lived in Tennessee since then. After more than almost four decades in America, I believe I also know my adopted country and the mindset of its citizens. Americans born here assume they know the Middle East and how to amicably deal with its inhabitants. Unfortunately, this is simply not the case. U.S. government policy toward the nations of the Middle East seems to be regressing rather than progressing, going backward instead of forward.

Policy-makers think they can solve the problems of the Middle East the way they have solved problems in the industrialized West. Government officials have obviously not studied the history, culture and religions of the region. They have failed to use the expertise and advice of Middle Easterners who live in America and abroad. Instead, academics from Harvard and Stanford, who acquire all their knowledge of that part of the world from books, are consulted by the U.S. government. It's not an exaggeration to say that any U.S.-based layman originally from the Middle East could give our government more effective advice.

Prior to World War II, after the collapse of the Ottoman Empire which ended its hegemony over the Middle East at the end of the first world war, the United States and Britain forced their political will on the Arab population. During the Versailles Peace Conference after World War I,

Über-colonialist Winston Churchill arbitrarily drew the lines on the map that crammed such disparate peoples as Shiites, Sunnis and Kurds into what became present-day Iraq, later calling it the worst blunder of his political life. (Actually, his invasion of Gallipoli in Turkey in 1915 was an even worse blooper, but that's a debate for another book.)

The West not only made disastrous cartographical decisions in the region, it also imposed unwanted rulers to protect its interests on these newly created nations, such as the Shah of Iran, King Faisal II of Iraq, King Fouad and his son, Farouk, of Egypt, and the reactionary royal family of Saudi Arabia. This high-handed treatment created raging resentment and resistance and generated the extremist ideology that still poisons the region to this day.

Imperialist interference, however, predates the post-World War I era. In 1882 the British invaded Egypt to crush a pro-democracy revolt against the Sultan of Egypt and his tyrannical taxes and remained there for decades, not leaving until 1956. In reaction to this egregious example of European colonialism, the radical Muslim Brotherhood came into being in 1919, the first of many terrorist groups to infest the Middle East. The Brotherhood unsuccessfully tried to oust the British occupiers and depose the hated royal family. In 1952, General Gamal Abdul Nasser achieved one of the Muslim Brotherhood's objectives and deposed the sybaritic King Farouk, ending the monarchy. In 1956, he again succeeded where the Brotherhood had failed and ended Britain's control of the Suez Canal.

But inarguably the worst example for Arabs of imperious meddling in Middle Eastern affairs by the West was the United Nations' approval of the creation of the state of Israel in 1948. The British were enraged by the U.N.'s decision, but acceded to its demand and withdrew from Israel/Palestine in a snit. Into this lacuna [or vacuum?] of foreign influence, the U.S. happily stepped in to protect the Jewish citizens of Israel. As Alexander Pope said, where angels fear to tread, fools … etc.

The American intrusion into Palestinian affairs has enraged the Muslim world ever since and among many, many other repercussions, fueled Osama bin Laden's psychotic decision to massacre almost 3,000 American innocents. (Bin Laden, however, shares most Muslims' resentment of foreign occupation of Muslim territory by "infidels," i.e., non-Muslims, and an even more compelling motivation for launching 9/11 was his rage over the stationing of American troops in the birthplace of Islam, Saudi Arabia, after Saddam Hussein invaded Kuwait in 1990.

(Muslims are so xenophobic, infidels are not even allowed to enter Mecca, although a handful Westerners, like 19th century British explorer Sir Richard Burton, have sneaked into the sacred city.)

Super sensitized by a millennium and a half of foreign domination dating back to the Byzantine and Ottoman empires, Muslim culture hellaciously resents occupation by non-Muslim powers. During the Six-Day War in 1967, Israel occupied Palestinian-controlled East Jerusalem and took possession of Islam's third holiest site, the Al-Aqsa Mosque. Israeli control of the revered shrine has been a twisting knife in the back of Muslims and one of the many reasons Middle Easterners abhor Israel and its primary patron, the U.S.

It's become a truism that the enmity between the West and Islamic nations will never end until the Israeli-Palestinian conflict is resolved. Until the Palestinians regain control of Al-Aqsa and secure self-rule over a portion of East Jerusalem, the problem will remain intractable.

Yet another source of Muslim rage is Israel's treatment of its Palestinian population as second-class citizens, with substandard housing and schools, inequity of income and so many other abuses that former President Jimmy Carter in his 2006 book, *Palestine Peace Not Apartheid*, alone among all other American politicians and statesmen, had the reckless temerity to call Israeli policy in the West Bank by its true name, *apartheid*. For this, American supporters of Israel called the 2002 Nobel Peace Prize winner a "racist" and "anti-Semite."

One of the call to arms during the American Revolution was "taxation without representation is unjust." When actress Vanessa Redgrave had the suicidal nerve to call Zionism implicitly racist because Israel taxes residents of the West Bank but denies them seats in its Knesset or parliament, she was labeled an anti-Semite and her once prosperous film career in America virtually evaporated.

The Muslim world considers the United States a biased agent representing Israeli, not Arab interests. No matter how well-intentioned and how hard the U.S. government tries to help Middle Eastern nations, they don't believe the U.S. is in their corner. They resent the fact that the American government tends to take the side of Israel against the Palestinians. (For the past 50 years, Israel has been the single largest recipient of U.S. economic and military aid, although in defense of our government's foreign policy, it should be noted that the second largest beneficiary of American largesse is Egypt, which may be its reward for being the only Arab country to sign a peace treaty with Israel.) Even so, the U.S. has never taken an even-handed approach to the Israeli-Palestinian quagmire.

The only American president Muslims have trusted since the founding of Israel in 1948 was Jimmy Carter. That's why Carter was able to win the acquiescence of Egypt and negotiate the Camp David Accords of 1978–1979. The Accords represent a rare achievement in Carter's otherwise failed presidency. (He regularly ranks near the bottom of lists of most effective American presidents, just above Herbert Hoover and Warren G. Harding!)

If Carter had won reelection in 1980, he probably would have secured another peace treaty between Israel and the rest of the Arab world.

Although not as much as they did Carter, Middle Easterners also trusted President Bill Clinton, and that may explain his success with the Oslo Accords in 1993 between Israeli Prime Minister Itzak Rabin and Palestinian President Yassir Arafat. In 2000 during the last year of the Clinton Administration, the two sides were tantalizingly close to a final agreement between Israeli Prime Minister Ehud Barak and Arafat.

The following Republican administration has been a disaster in achieving peace between Israel and the Palestinians because Muslims consider Republicans anti-Arab and arrogant and so they do not trust or respect any dovish recommendations from Bush and Co.

The most important—and intractable—problem in the Middle East remains the irreconcilable aspirations of the Palestinians and Israelis. The U.S. government should treat both sides even-handedly and act as an unbiased broker to bring peace to the entire region. If after five more years of fruitless negotiations, Israel and the Palestinians still not have reached a permanent accord, the U.S., as bitter a pill as this will be, will have to withdraw its influence from that region and stop interfering in Middle Eastern affairs.

The U.S. must stop supplying all assistance, including money and weapons, to any nation in the region. Our government has had more than half a century to end this endless crisis, and other countries should be given a crack at solving the insoluble.

Another problem created by the U.S. is its meddling in the affairs of the oil-producing nations of the Middle East. These governments are corrupt, zealous and anti-democratic, and yet because they sit on one-third of the world's oil wealth, they are treated by us as friends, even though polls show that 70 percent of Saudi Arabians want American troops out of their country and admit that they believe it is morally justifiable to kill Americans. (As it has been endlessly reported, 18 of the 19 9/11 hijackers came from Saudi Arabia.) We need to withdraw our tentacles from Kuwait, Saudi Arabia, Pakistan and every other nation in the Muslim world, and let them know we are not going to bother them, so stop bothering us.

If their *jihad* against the West does not end after we leave the region, we will return and destroy their infrastructure as we have already trashed Afghanistan's and Iraq's. There should be no American military presence in the Middle East period. Terrorists should be warned that if they continue their murderous assaults on the Western democracies, they do so at their own peril. We can continue to exchange students and have cultural intercourse with the Arab world, but only if they continue their good behavior. The threat of punishment must be credible, but limited to aerial bombardment and no commitment or waste of American military lives. We won't invade you as we fruitlessly did in Iraq, we will just make good on the threat made against North Vietnam during the 1960s and 70s: our Air Force will bomb you back into the Stone Age, where your ethics and violent tendencies already reside. Then we will leave the region to its sanguine fate and self-immolation.

Muslims are compulsive fighters. Their religion encourages aggressive, brave behavior with the promise of instant access to paradise in return for their martyrdom. It was this promise that allowed a tiny group of Bedouin brigands to conquer an empire larger than ancient Rome's within a century of their emergence from the dusty boondocks of the Arabian peninsula beginning in the seventh century.

The solipsistic mistake of America and the rest of the industrialized West has always been their attempt to change the moral and political philosophy of Muslims. For more than a century, well-meaning but misguided colonial powers have tried to force democracy on inherently repressive regimes and peoples who have no respect or interest in adopting democratic ideals. This colonial mindset on the part of Britain and France after the first world war arbitrarily redrew the maps of areas that became present-day Syria, Lebanon, Palestine, Iraq, Jordan and Kuwait, and forced ethnic and religious groups who had been enemies for centuries to cohabit the same artificially created countries that have led to the internecine bloodbaths in Lebanon and the Kurdish regions of Turkey, among others, that continue to rage to the present day.

History has taught us that people will not change their ways and politics by foreign coercion. As in Europe in centuries past, warring entities within countries split amoeba-like, reunited, split again and finally reunited for good after conflicts of *self*-determination such as the War of the Roses in 15th century England, the same nation's Civil War in the mid-17th, the religious wars that savaged and depopulated what eventually became Germany in the 16th and 17th centuries, the royalist and civil wars that convulsed Spain in the 19th and 20th centuries, the *Risorgimento*, Italy's wars of unification, in the 19th century, as well as the ethnic/religious conflicts that are still fueled by Basque separatists in Spain, the French and Flemish speaking peoples of Belgium, and "The Troubles" in Northern Ireland that after 40 years and 2,000 civilian deaths later at last seem to be coming to an end—the latter a paradigm for a foreign "occupier's" (Britain's) failure to impose a peace that only now seems achievable because the indigenous Protestants and Catholics have grown tired of fighting due to old age and have lost the aggressive tendencies of youth. (The real reason crime has decreased in the United States is not due to more policing or stiffer sentencing, but the simple demographic fact that the Baby Boom generation is nearing retirement age and statistically most crimes are committed by twentysomethings, an ever dwindling portion of the U.S. population.)

A Prognosis and Prescription for the Middle East Mess

To recap, which is necessary, because the screed above needs to be repeated over and over again until it finally lodges itself in the consciousness of the inattentive folks who run this country, we have inhabited the worst of all possible worlds with our meddling in the affairs of Middle Eastern nations during the last century and this one with use of military force, the viscerally resented occupation of Muslim territory, oppression, and the support of corrupt dictators loathed by their repressed populations.

The West's misguided policies have given birth to extremist movements like the Muslim Brotherhood in Egypt, the *fedayeen*, the Al-Aqsa Martyrs' Brigade and Hamas in Palestine, the Islamo-fascist theocracy of Iran, Al Qaeda in Saudi Arab, Afghanistan and Pakistan, Hezbollah in Lebanon, and most recently the Muqtada al-Sadr's Mahdi death squads in Iraq.

The only reasonable and effective solution is for the nations of the industrialized West, mainly the United States and the United Kingdom, to withdraw its military forces from that part of the world completely, and end our direct and indirect involvement in the entire Muslim world.

The United States and European nations must struggle even harder than they have in the past to end the conflict between Israel and its subject Palestinian population before we depart the region, but regardless of whether peace is eventually achieved, we must leave sooner rather than later. If the warring sides do not accept American peace proposals, we must leave them to their fate, even if it results in civil wars throughout the region, because the current situation in Israel already approximates civil war and the conflict in Iraq constitutes one.

That recommendation may sound like a cruel and harsh application of *Realpolitik*, but the alternative is the continued waste of American lives and financial resources. The presence of Western influence in the Middle East usually aggravates the problem; the nations in the region must be allowed self-determination in reaching a peaceful settlement without outside intervention or influence. At the risk of sounding isolationist, and frankly I don't believe there's anything wrong with isolationism, the United States simply doesn't have the power or influence to be the world's policeman.

Beyond the Middle East

Only the most obtuse political observers can have failed to notice that during the past six years of the current administration, our relationships with the rest of the world have shamefully deteriorated compared to the past.

Our foreign policy has been so off-putting, unilateralist and arrogant that even our once friendly European allies regularly denounce the United States in their legislatures and media. Our image abroad has been trashed, and we have lost both the respect and even admiration of our foreign friends and the fear of our foes.

Cowboy diplomacy has brought us to this untenable position, just as gunboat diplomacy during America's colonialist/imperialist era in the 19th and early 20th centuries poisoned our relationships with out-gunned and out-manned Third World countries. (Reference Cuba, the Philippines, the domination of most of Central America by United Fruit, which imposed and deposed dictators in that region at will, and the overthrow of Hawaii's last royal ruler by the American Dole family's pineapple company.)

The chief reason for the deterioration of America's image abroad is, of course, our disastrous adventure in Iraq. Post 9/11 but pre-Iraq, most of the world shared our sense of loss of almost 3,000 New Yorkers and supported our response to the tragedy by invading Al Qaeda's spider hole, Afghanistan, so enthusiastically that a large number of European nations contributed troops to the incursion.

Afghanistan, like World War II, was deemed a "good war." Iraq, like Vietnam, is beyond bad. In contrast, most of Europe denounced our entry into Iraq, most notably Germany and France, and immediately rejected our spurious justifications for taking on Saddam Hussein just as much later most Americans and their elected representatives have come to do. Only the United Kingdom—along with much smaller participation by Spain, Canada and Australia—joined us in our folly, and the U.S. and the

U.K. supplied 90 to 95 percent of the troops sent to Iraq, despite President Bush's and his neocon cronies' delusional claim that a "coalition" of many countries had contributed military aid and manpower.

Most European nations immediately recognized the lunacy of attacking a country—no matter how psychopathic its leader—that posed no strategic threat to the United States or the rest of the West. Although forensic psychologists have used the same diagnosis—"malign narcissist"—to describe Saddam that they have applied to Stalin and Hitler, but the world is filled with such lethal narcissistic strongmen, and we can't overthrow all of them. Again, America is not an international cop. Tragically, it took American voters three years to catch up with that European *aperçu*.

U.S. leaders further inflamed European complaints by denouncing those nations, especially France and Germany—the latter once our most enthusiastic ally on the continent. Most infamously, former Secretary of Defense Donald H.Rumsfeld dismissed France and Germany in an embarrassing example of ugly Americanism as "Old Europe," to which French President Jacques Chirac responded in *Parlement*, "We are an *ancient* nation." ("*Nous sommes un regime ancien.*")

French public pinion was again enraged by photos and videotape of Americans pouring French wine in the gutter and threatening to stop all French luxury imports to the U.S.

Prior to March 20, 2003, when American troops crossed the Kuwaiti border into Iraq, the U.S. was a prestigious, not to mention the only, remaining superpower in the world, which enthusiastically supported our involvement in Serbia, Bosnia Herzegovina, Afghanistan, Grenada to rescue American medical students who didn't need rescuing, and Panama to oust narcotrafficking strongman Manuel Noriega.

The United States remains a superpower, but a superpower in decline and disgrace.

Fear and Loathing in the Rest of the World

Contempt for America is not exclusive to Europe. Another region of the world that resents and even loathes us as much as Middle Easterners do is Latin America. The origins of that loathing predate U.S. meddling in the

Muslim world by more than 100 years, when at the end of the Mexican-American War in 1848, the U.S. annexed more than half of Mexico's territory as its booty for winning the conflict, although the U.S. paid Mexico $15 million for its larceny and forgave $3.25 in debt Mexico owed American citizens. The U.S. may have been an aggressive imperialist power, but it was also a generous imperialist power.

Also in the mid-19th century, an American mercenary, William Walker, with the backing of shipping and railroad magnate Cornelius Vanderbilt invaded not one but three Latin American countries—Mexico, Honduras and Nicaragua, and in the latter set himself up as its President and reinstated slavery there.

The U.S.'s voracious land grabs continued and by the end of the 19th century, after its victory during the Spanish-American War, it annexed Cuba, Puerto Rico (not to mention halfway around the world the Philippines.) In 1916, the U.S. resumed its meddling in Mexico when President Woodrow Wilson sent 150,000 members of the American Expeditionary Force under General "Black Jack" Pershing into that country to capture *bandito* or revolutionary (depending on one's position on the liberal/conservative spectrum) Pancho Villa after his brigands massacred 17 residents of Columbus, New Mexico. American corporations' high-handed interference in Central America and the Caribbean in the 20th century.

The United States' failure to oust Cuba's Fidel Castro during the Bay of Pigs fiasco in 1961 began an enmity toward America, which with the further irritation of economic sanctions and risible attempts by the CIA and the Mafia to off the Cuban dictator with Bugs Bunny vs. Elmer Fudd-type weapons such as exploding cigars, continues to this day. In general, the U.S. has tended to favor the rich, reactionary ruling classes in this part of the world at the expense of the poor. During the Cold War, America's leaders didn't care how corrupt or repressive Latin American dictators were as long as they shared our paranoid hatred of Marxism and the Soviet Union, including the much-loathed General Augusto Pinochet of Chile, who was accused of murdering 3,100 political dissidents, torturing tens of thousands more and exiling hundreds of thousands during his 17-year dictatorship.

The most recent example of how U.S. support of the rich over the poor is neo-Marxist Venezuelan President Hugo Chavez, who abhors us with the same passion our government has hated Castro for more than 40 years to such an extent that he had allied himself with Saddam Hussein and Libya's Moammar Gadhafi.

After the fall of the Soviet Union and the end of its financial and military support of the Castro regime, our continued opposition to that country's leader is puzzling and inexplicable. Cuba is an exhausted and bankrupt nation that poses no threat to anyone except perhaps its own citizens, who endure on a subsistence level, not only due to Castro's discredited Marxist policies but also because of our own decades of economic sanctions against the island, which only hurt its people, not its necrotic leader, reports of whose imminent death, as Mark Twain said about himself, have been "greatly exaggerated." Castro's ability to hold on to power, not to mention life, recalls the 1970s joke about the Spanish dictator's lingering on earth: "Is Franco still dead?"

The actual reason sanctions remain in place is not our fear of a Marxist regime in this hemisphere or even Castro's grotesque violation of human rights. Archconservative upper-class Cuban-Americans who fled their homeland after Castro came to power in 1959 and left their wealth behind have held on to their blind rage against the tyrant who dispossessed them. Whenever Anglo-Congressional members suggest even the slightest easing of American restrictions against Cuba, the Cuban-American lobby seems to have post-traumatic stress syndrome-like flashbacks to their flight from Cuba in the early 1960s, and quash any Congressional efforts to improve relations with their homeland.

Sanctions are not only ineffective—Castro remains in power despite decades of their imposition—they are self-defeating for American policy goals. Rather than contributing to the ouster of the rulers of repressive regime, sanctions have the converse, ironic effect of strengthening these criminal strongmen. When the U.S. government imposes sanctions that economically hurt the citizens of these regimes, their leaders denounce American "cruelty," and the people rally behind these dictators as heroes for standing up against the Yanquis.

Due to effective censorship of the foreign media (during Saddam Hussein's tenure, Iraqis were not even allowed access to the liberating and informative influence of the Internet), the people in these countries remain ignorant of their leaders' corruption, mismanagement and obscene, luxury-filled lives. While sanctions impoverish citizens, dictators enjoy black-market fueled extravagances and perks. Saddam built dozens of palaces while his people lived in crumbling homes with ever deteriorating infrastructure. The average family during Saddam's tenure was so poor that it could only afford to eat chicken once a month.

While North Korea's demented, misnamed "dear leader," Kim Jong-Il, fancies Cuban cigars, caviar, Courvoisier (Napoleon's favorite cognac too) and a fleet of imported luxury automobiles Jerry Seinfeld might envy, his citizens are literally starving to death, forced to eat grass to fill their empty, bloated bellies. The increased power that sanctions provided dictators allowed them to jail even more dissidents for pro-democracy "crimes" and criticism of human rights violations because the majority of the population supported their leaders due to their anti-American rants.

The U.S. government is justified in its loathing of these repressive regimes, but their method of dealing with them should be passive rather than aggressive. These dictators have an inferiority complex, and the best way to handle them is by ignoring and isolating them. If we disapprove of human rights abusers, we should ignore them, not sanction them, isolate them diplomatically. America should only engage in offensive tactics if it is directly or indirectly threatened, such as invading Afghanistan in response to 9/11 or attacking Libya in 1986 after its leader, Moammar Gadhafi, whose erratic and self-sabotaging behavior some have theorized was fueled by methamphetamine abuse, bombed a nightclub in Germany frequented by American G.I.s and even more egregiously was implicated in the 1988 downing of Pan Am Flight 103 over Lockerbie, Scotland.

To show repressive regimes American willingness to reward good behavior, the leaders and citizens of small, democratic countries should be feted with kindness, respect and increased financial assistance. We should learn more about their problems so we can help solve them. We need to devote more of our resources to regions in our own hemisphere, like Latin

America, and spend less on those further away. Benevolent American diplomacy may not change the mindset of dictators, but their citizens may get the message of the United States' good intentions and ability to improve their standard of living and promote civil rights to the extent that they eventually rise up and boot their noxious leaders out of office. If neither dictators nor their suffering people respond to our example, we must simply cut our losses as we also must do in the Middle East if our peace-making efforts continue to fail, and leave our unfortunate neighbors to the south to their undeserved fate.

CHAPTER FIVE

Saving America's Healthcare System

The unwritten social contract, to borrow Rousseau's term, between every nation and its citizens is the obligation to provide free and quality education for their children, afford protection against crime and environmental hazards, prevent domestic and overseas terrorist attacks and offer affordable health insurance for all—the latter the focus of this chapter.

Good health is not a luxury, it is one of the inalienable rights our Founding Fathers neglected to mention in the Declaration of Independence where it says that all men are entitled to "life, liberty and the pursuit of happiness"—neglected probably because in the late 18th century healthcare was provided by charlatans and quacks and its effectiveness so poor to non-existent (leeches! blood-letting! emetic and rectal purges!), that medical treatment seemed more like a curse than inalienable right. Until the beginning of the 20th century and the introduction of internal surgery, hospitalization was a one-way trip patients took en route to the morgue.

Today, with the miracle advances of high-tech medicine that increase lifespan and remission rates, it is the duty of the government to provide every citizen with access to life-saving treatment. Adequate healthcare is a right, not a luxury, but a right the poor and an ever-increasing percentage of the middle class do not enjoy as an unacceptable 48 million Americans, among them 9 million children—a disgrace that marks us as the only industrialized nation guilty of such a tear in the social safety net—do not have health insurance and the number of uninsured continues to increase every two to three years by another five million. Fortunately, these unfortunates don't die, they end up at substandard a.k.a. charity hospitals for the indigent.

You don't have to be a jingoist to maintain that the United States is the greatest, richest country in the world, and spends more money providing healthcare for its citizens than any other industrialized nation. The reputation of American medicine's excellence is so well-known that ailing people from all over the world come here to access it.

It's a little known fact that whenever Mother Teresa became ill, she didn't tough it out in one of her non-tech hospices in Calcutta, but flew to New York to receive treatment by America's best and brightest medical practitioners, according to a BBC documentary entitled "Holy Cow." Ditto the Shah of Iran and every infirm member of the Saudi royal family. For the very best in cardiovascular treatment, Baylor University in Houston, Texas, with its superstar heart surgeon, Dr. Michael DeBakey, was a medical tourist's luxury destination in the 1970s and '80s. In fact, DeBakey was an intimate of the late King of Saudi Arabia, probably because the doctor cut open the king so many times. The Cleveland Clinic, the Mayo Clinic and Johns Hopkins University are other popular magnets for the foreign elite seeking state-of-the-art medical treatment.

And yet despite physicians like DeBakey's availability to well-insured natives and well-heeled foreigners, when it comes to the average quality of healthcare in America, the nation ranks No. 37, approximately the same position as Puerto Rico and some Third World countries. In the same ranking, most European nations enjoy a two-digit lead over the United States.

The quality or mediocrity of U.S. healthcare is directly related to the socio-economic status of the patient—a phenomenon that Marx should rise from the grave and take a bow for because of his condemnation of the inequity of the distribution of wealth in the world of capitalism and everything it can buy, including a competent doctor. The top segment of the

American population, the rich, have superb health insurance and receive superb healthcare. The middle class, which continues to slip down the economic ladder as wages fail to keep pace with inflation, have mediocre health insurance and endure mediocre healthcare. They have more out-of-pocket medical expenses due to stratospheric co-payments, sky-high deductibles, prescription drug costs that constitute blatant gouging by Big Pharm, and premiums that insurance companies have been known to double arbitrarily from year to year without blushing.

Employees lucky enough to have their insurance premiums partially subsidized by employers have to pay even higher premiums if family members also need coverage. The middle class is going broke paying for health insurance—when they can even get it. If you have a pre-existing condition, you are *persona non grata* and dead meat as far as insurance carriers are concerned.

Then there's the tragedy of the bottom segment of the population, both the unemployed and even the working poor, who typically have no private insurance. The rich and middle class ignore the plight of these poor at their own economic peril because they end up indirectly paying for the medical care of the uninsured. (Unlike in some parts of the Third World, where the underclass are allowed to die for lack of treatment—hence the "popularity" of such places as Mother Teresa's hospices *cum* morgues in India, the U.S. government, despite its callous indifference to so much other suffering endured by its *lumpen* proletariat, isn't quite heartless enough to let its most unfortunate citizens die in the street like dogs as they literally do in many parts of the underdeveloped world.

(There is a ghastly website which I have stopped visiting because it's too heart-breaking to watch, where a light blinks every few seconds, with each twinkling star representing a terminal child in a poor nation who has just expired. The lights on the maps of India and China are as bright as Times Square's.)

Without health insurance, the poor can't afford to see a private primary care physician or family doctor, so they wait until they are severely ill and seek treatment at the emergency rooms of hospitals, which are required by law to treat the uninsured regardless of their ability to pay. Treatment is free for the indigent, but the rich and middle class pick up the tab, as the hospital passes the unreimbursed costs on to its insurance carriers, who in turn pass them on to their insurees in the form of higher premiums, co-pays and deductibles.

One of the reasons emergency room treatment is so much more expensive than a trip to the family doctor is that poor people without insurance cannot afford to have routine checkups when they go to the emergency room because they are in the advanced stages of their illness. Regular visits to a primary care physician provide prophylactic procedures that stop illnesses before they start, ongoing treatment for hypertension and other heart disease, kidney ailments, which when untreated require expensive dialysis sooner than the insured lucky enough to have preventive treatment, the lack of which can also lead to severe complications from diabetes and cardiovascular disease. Also, the ER doctor has to do a battery of tests, evaluate the patient from A to Z. ER fees are usually higher because the room is filled with advanced equipment, especially in big hospitals.

Non-emergency room hospital care for the uninsured also ends up costing the rich and middle classes, whose higher insurance premiums subsidize the poor. A study that appeared in the journal *Health Affairs* on May 8, 2007, made front page news across the country when it revealed that hospitals charge uninsured patients 2 ½ times more than the privately insured, and three times more than Medicare pays for its enrollees. *Health Affairs* reported that the uninsured are billed—but do not pay—full price while those with private insurance and Medicare recipients enjoy dramatic discounts.

As an example, the medical journal said a hospital might bill $12,500 for an appendectomy, but accept only a fraction of that charge, $5,000, from private carriers. And patients with private insurance pay only a fraction of that fraction thanks to low co-pays and/or deductibles. Private insurers are able to pay less because they enjoy the leverage of being able to send large numbers of their members to hospitals, which accept the reduced fee because bulk compensates for lower reimbursement.

The poor and uninsured aren't really getting ripped off by hospitals that charge them full price because they simply default on their payments, although some for-profit hospitals are notorious for aggressively recouping their costs from the working poor by garnishing their already subsistence-level wages. Gerard F. Anderson, a research scientist at Johns Hopkins University who wrote the *Health Affairs* article, believes hospitals are gouging the nation's most vulnerable citizens. "Hospitals shouldn't be charging three times [Medicare rates], especially from poor people who are uninsured," Anderson told the *Los Angeles Times*.

This loony billing system antagonizes everyone—the rich, the middle class, the poor, hospitals and insurance providers. It's an equal opportunity aggravator. Insurers complain because of the rising cost of new, high-tech medical procedures. Healthcare providers, both doctors and hospitals, complain about decreasing profits due to decreasing reimbursement by insurance carriers and the torturous paperwork and regulations government bureaucrats force them to accept in return for reimbursing their treatment of Medicare and Medicaid recipients. Employers are frustrated because insurers keep increasing the cost of covering their employees, and employees are panic-stricken because employers sometimes raise their share of the premium cost so extortionately—sometimes doubling premiums or deductibles in a single year—that workers end up dropping their coverage because they simply can't afford to pay.

The system is fatigued and broken. When the government makes cosmetic changes like requiring Medicaid to lower its payment to providers, the federal and state bureaucracies think they are improving the situation but are actually exacerbating it. Providers believe they can solve their financial problems by demanding higher reimbursement from the government, which with the current tight-fisted Republican administration, ain't gonna happen.

The foundation of the nation's medical structure is crumbling like a moldy ante bellum mansion and will soon collapse. Despite the panacea promised by Medicare Plan D's prescription drug program, the plan incorporates the infamous "doughnut," which stiffs enrollees after their prescription costs reach a certain amount and reimbursement isn't reinstated until a few thousand more dollars in bills accrue, the cost of which has to be borne by Plan D beneficiaries. Plus, the plan is the handiwork of anal-retentive federal bureaucrats who seem congenitally incapable of creating simple, easy to understand and follow regulations that must be heeded by pharmacies that expect reimbursement for the cost of their customers' drugs. Each state in the country has up to 20 different coverage plans, which confuse recipients and generate even more burdensome paperwork for pharmacies.

Everyone is a villain of this piece; there are no innocent bystanders.

No. 1: Hospitals set extortionate prices that amount to gouging, like charging $30 for a syringe that costs them a buck fifty, reminiscent of the Pentagon's infamous $800 toilet seats and $500 hammers. Sometimes, hospital billing practices are worse than gouging and constitute outright fraud. They pay their "chiefs" (hospital executives) obscenely inflated salaries á la Wall Street's overcompensated CEOS and remunerate their "Indians" (rank and file employees like nurses and orderlies) substandard wages. Hospitals further exacerbate the cost of doing business by offering expensive gimmicks such as "health fairs" where they visit shopping malls and monitor blood pressure and prescreen for colon and breast cancer and diabetes as a way of luring patients to their establishments.

Hospitals too often seem more concerned about increasing their profit margins rather than the quality of patient care. Heartless hospitals and insurers eject patients prematurely (the average post-natal hospital stay of mothers over the years has declined from an average of two days to the bum's rush of only one). Medicare patients are also kicked out by hospitals early because Medicare pays the same amount per diagnoses called DRGs whether the patient is hospitalized for one or 10 days. Greed forces patients to go home earlier than it is safe to do so, which may result in complications and rehospitalization, adding even more to the cost of healthcare. Another cost-cutting dodge by hospitals is decreasing the nurse/patient ratio, which causes patient dissatisfaction and frustration due to less than prompt responses by overworked nurses, who at the end of the day are miserable and exhausted by their increased work load.

No. 2: Private insurers are just as culpable for the medical mess the U.S. is mired in as hospitals. Reimbursements for identical services are arbitrary and vary from carrier to carrier. Blue Cross may pay hospitals $1,000 for an appendectomy, while Aetna bills $1,500.

You don't have to be a member of the lunatic left to characterize the profits of insurance companies as obscene. Their revenue is so high because among other practices they charge administrative fees ranging from 20 to 25 percent, while Medicare, a rare example of federal government efficiency, has costs roughly around three percent. Every year, for the same health plans, private insurance companies raise their premiums and further fatten their coffers with the dodge of increasing the deductible to the point where employers and employees have to drop their coverage because they can't afford deductibles that can climb to such middle-class budget-busting prices as $1,000 to $7,000 per year. Another insurance company dodge that has resulted in hundreds of class action lawsuits is the flat-out fraudulent practice of automatically refusing reimbursement on the first request for payment, and the time devoted to second and even third resubmissions enrage patients and add to the costs incurred by doctors and hospitals, which have to hire additional staff to handle the extra paperwork. Already enjoying huge profits, when their revenues shrink just a bit, insurance companies spike their premiums extortionately and make even more money.

No. 3: Doctors also belong on the miscreants list. One of the reasons besides pricier medical innovations that the cost of healthcare has far outpaced the rate of inflation over the past few decades are that there is now a surplus of physicians compared to the past. Newly minted doctors emerge from medical school burdened with monstrous student loans that range between $100,000 and $200,000 and monthly repayment charges often approximate the cost of a home mortgage. All these aggressive "surplus" doctors compete for a bigger share of the same amount of funding. We also have more subspecialized doctors than primary care physicians. Subspecialized doctors use more medical and surgical high-tech procedures, which are more expensive than practicing generic medicine, which was done by general practitioners in the 1970s and early 80s treating high blood pressure, diabetes, common colds and pneumonia.

Preventive medicine may be used more widely now than in the past, e.g., colonoscopies, mammograms, etc. Defensive medicine prompted by the increasing number of malpractice suits by ambulance-chasing lawyers can make medicine more expensive. All of the above are not necessarily the fault of doctors, but when you have more doctors on the block, many of them have to repay expensive student loans incurred by their medical school education. This encourages them to do unnecessary and frequent procedures. Some may order more expensive tests, while simple cheaper tests can give the same results. Probably, this practice arises from ignorance or over diagnosis. Sometimes, incentives from diagnostic institutions for doctors to refer patients to these institutions for X-ray and other testing. Although such practices are illegal according to Stark's Law, which prohibits the referral of patients in return for monetary gain.

Other things may be done by some doctors unwisely such as prescribing expensive drugs, which could be replaced with cheaper generics. This may be done out of ignorance or due to incentives from drug companies.

Sometimes general practitioners and others perform unnecessary tests on every patient who walks into their office as a source of revenue, e.g., EKGs, heart stress tests and bone scans to check women for osteoporosis.

In general, doctors need to be thrifty and knowledgeable when ordering tests or prescribing medicine. They need to use expensive high-tech procedures only as necessary to meet the standards of healthcare set the local community and the United States. Sometimes if these tests are not done, as indicated, the physician may be liable to malpractice suits.

Another problem with doctors is the unfair distinctions made between one form of specialization and another, e.g. anesthesia vs. internal medicine. The pay scale per unit of time is out of proportion, which makes some physicians resentful. Also, the decrease in reimbursement by the government and insurance companies discourage prospective doctors from entering the medical field.

No. 4: Patients are not innocent bystanders either and contribute to the unnecessary rise in the cost of healthcare. Their expectations are high, and they demand more and more services. Terminally ill patients with a very poor prognosis for survival are kept alive needlessly at the insistence of loved ones, who demand that their dying relatives remain in intensive care units to do everything possible but not necessarily helpful, including ventilators and dialysis. They receive expensive antibiotics and heart medications, as well as remaining connected to multiple tubes despite the fact that the terminally ill patient is brain-dead and has advanced multi-organ failure. These patients often linger for months and months even though they have basically become vegetables, and after hundreds of thousands of dollars are spent on heroic preservation efforts, they die anyway. Many times families want their loved ones kept alive to continue to collect the patients' Social Security payments.

(Former socialite and philanthropist Sunny von Bülow, whose husband Claus was convicted but later acquitted after a retrial for overdosing his wife with insulin, has remained in a persistent vegetative state with no hope of revival since 1981 in a pricey private hospital room with round-the-clock nursing care simply because she's the heiress to a $70-million public utilities fortune and can afford it—or at least her two children can.

(Terri Schiavo's irrational parents refused to pull her feeding tube for the 15 years she spent in a persistent vegetative coma on the public tab until her husband Michael took his in-laws to court. Her wide-open eyes and smile fooled her parents for years even though tests showed that she was brain-dead and unaware of her surroundings.)

Millions more are wasted on "preemies," premature babies with terminal neurological disorders, underdeveloped hearts and missing brain parts. Understandably, the distraught mother of an impaired newborn is incapable of making a rational cost/benefit ratio evaluation and insists that her infant receive useless, high-tech medical intervention that may prolong life but not save it.

Nonagenarians with one foot already in the grave are put on artificial life support to prolong their lives. Transplant surgeries are performed on old, low prognosis patients (i.e., very short life expectancies) suffering from chronic serious diseases and other unsurvivable illnesses. Bereaved family members insist on keeping relatives on expensive life support even when their life expectancy may be as short as six months. (In 1995, baseball Hall of Famer Mickey Mantle, despite a 43-year history of alcoholism, hepatitis C and a hepatoma (tumor) which should have disqualified him, received a liver transplant anyway … and died three months later.

In the 1970s, healthcare providers were more rational, although emotional critics would call them heartless, and refused to provide critical life support and transplants for patients over 65. Now everyone qualifies for expensive and heroic preservation efforts regardless how quixotic—even for patients in their eighties and nineties. Such efforts can be made for those between ages 65 and 90 based on common sense.

The money spent on these lost souls siphons off the limited pool of healthcare funds, which could be put to much better use treating less severely ill patients. We could save hundreds of thousands of these salvageable people, using the money saved for preventive treatment of children, adults and seniors with a good chance of survival.

Many less ill patients also abuse the system, and instead of making an appointment with their primary care physician, who will charge them for treatment, they turn up at emergency rooms in the middle of the night suffering from coughs and the common cold because they don't have to pay. Indeed, mind-blowingly, colds are the No. 1 cause of ER visits. (The much more serious affliction of irritable bowel syndrome is second.)

More waste: battery-powered chairs are used by patients with legitimate mobility problems, but their friends see them scooting around the neighborhood like superannuated Hell's Angels, and then they want a chair for themselves even though they can get around on their own without spiffy wheels, thank you very much.

Other patients want a motorized chair to lift them into the bathtub or their motor vans, and like the senior citizen bikers, they demand and get Medicare to pay for these costly machines. All this uninformed patient involvement contributes to the rise in healthcare costs, and patients are partially to blame.

No. 5: High Technology. There are some innocent, non-larcenous justifications for the rise in healthcare costs. Legitimate high-tech procedures also account for the increase. For example, invasive radiology, ultrasound and C-T scans, arrived on the scene in the late 1970s and early 1980s, while MRIs turned up in the late 1980s and early 1990s. Invasive radiology like angiography and angioplasty were only employed in teaching hospitals in the 1970s when they were still considered experimental procedures. Now their use is endemic.

Similarly, stents, which are plastic or metal tubes used to reopen collapsed or blocked arteries (Vice President Dick Cheney has had a zillion of these devices inserted in his atherosclerotic arteries), were only used to treat heart disease but now these expensive props are used for all vascular diseases. Endoscopy, in which a gastroenterologist sticks a tube with a tiny camera at its end up the patient's end, was primitive and rarely used in the 1970s, but now with easier to use flexible endoscopes, endoscopy is standard procedure used everywhere. Sometimes these procedures are frequently performed unnecessarily, and medical equipment manufacturers use costly promotional gimmicks like free "seminars" in Antigua and Bali to convince doctors to adopt them.

High-tech medicine is expensive, but it does add to the high quality of medical treatment in the United States by employing helpful tools to diagnose and treat patients. But if used extensively and unnecessarily, these procedures will increase the cost of healthcare enormously.

Manufacturers erroneously promise hospitals that the equipment will pay for itself in less than five years and offer the added incentive of reminding hospital administrators that private insurers and Medicare will pay for the devices anyway. These manufacturers aggressively promote their products to the providers.

No. 6: Big Pharm, a.k.a prescription drug manufacturers, also make the list of healthcare robber barons. There are too many drugs available for treating the same disease, including multiple brand names for identical group of drugs, for example blood pressure medications like ARBs, ACEIs and calcium channel blockers—all these medications—as many as six to eight brands—in each group of drugs are equally effective in treating the same medical problem. Different antibiotics are prescribed for the same bacterial infections. This duplication of effort is a result of too much competition between drug companies, although in the exact opposite of the classic economic theory that increased supply causes decreased prices, this competition does not reduce the cost of prescription drugs. To keep prices high, drug companies pressure providers—hospitals and physicians—to use their brand of a specific drug. So, if there are, for example, six different brands of the same group of drugs, they will be equally divided among patients. Because six drugs are available, profits are split six ways among drug companies. In order to keep profits high, manufacturers have to sell their products at six times the actual cost of producing the drugs.

To keep or increase their share of the profits, manufacturers have to spend more money on advertising in the form of free drug samples for doctors and even costlier TV advertising that seduces an uninformed public into demanding that their doctors prescribe the advertised brand. Some TV drug commercials are so devious, they don't even tell you the purpose of the drug that is being advertised and simply urge the layman viewer to "ask your doctor about …"

If legislation mandated that only one brand be made available for each disease, the brand would satisfy all patients who need the medication, and the result could be that prescriptions would cost only one-sixth of what they do compared to the current cornucopia of multiple, duplicative brands.

In the Third World and Europe, U.S. drug makers spend 20 percent less to market their products compared to their advertising budgets in the states. Canada is even more frugal and spends 50 percent less than drug companies do here. Canadians receive the same drug from the same drug company, but prices, which are set by the government, are much lower than in this country. To make up for their decrease in profits abroad, American drug manufacturers inflate the prices they charge their own citizens.

Taking a page from the manufacturers of medical equipment, drug companies also use promotional gimmicks such as small gifts, expensive dinners, "seminars" at luxury resorts around the world where doctors are actually paid a fee, euphemistically referred to as "honorariums," allegedly to compensate them for "advising" the companies on how to promote their drugs, even though the seminars at exotic locales, etc., show that the companies already know how to do so quite nicely. The consumer ends up paying for all these promotional gimmicks in the form of higher prices charged by drug manufacturers to finance the gimmicks.

No. 7: Malpractice attorneys, also known as ambulance-chasers and PI (personal injury) lawyers. Malpractice lawsuits, which often award millions if not billions of dollars to compensate plaintiffs who feel they are the victim of shoddy or incompetent medical care, increase the cost of healthcare because malpractice insurance carriers pass on the expense of litigation in the form of higher premiums for the insured and lower reimbursement for healthcare providers.

Abusive litigiousness also raises the cost of doctors' malpractice insurance premiums, which in the South have reached as high as $30,000 to $60,000 per year and $100,000 in California or New York, although years ago, the California legislature passed a law setting a cap on the amount of monetary awards for pain and suffering, which immediately made malpractice insurance less ruinous and more affordable in the state. Until it enacted similar caps, the state of Nevada suffered a doctor shortage crisis, especially among OB/GYN physicians, who found their sky-high premiums made it impossible to make a profit after spending as much as 90 percent of their income on malpractice insurance. Many physicians simply left the state.

Law schools churn out ever increasing numbers of lawyers, who are chasing the same amount of legal business that a smaller, previous generation of lawyers competed for, and in order to increase revenue, malpractice lawyers file even more lawsuits, further driving up the cost of provider's malpractice insurance. To avoid lawsuits, doctors end up practicing what is known as "defensive medicine," which consists of ordering extra and often unnecessary tests just to be sure that lawyers don't turn around and sue them for not performing those tests, which attorneys can then claim have caused their clients medical problems.

A Light at the End of the Tunnel of Runaway Insurance Costs and Unavailability

To recap, the current healthcare system in the U.S. is unfair, heterogeneous, i.e., each drug company arbitrarily charges providers different prices while coverage and premiums offered employers and the self-employed differ from plan to plan, with the self-employed being gouged even more than employers because the solo insurance consumer doesn't have the clout to negotiate lowers fees that employers with the ability to enroll huge numbers of employees can.

The complexity of Medicare, Medicaid, private health insurance and managed care or HMOs creates hassles and confusion, increasing the financial burden of the billing and collection departments of doctors and hospitals. Patients are frustrated because lay people often can't understand the difference between one insurance plan and another.

When Medicare's Prescription Drug Plan D was introduced in January 2006, so many insurance plans with different drugs allowed or prohibited on their formularies left beneficiaries of the new Medicare service so confused that they swamped the agency's telephone help lines, and some patients who couldn't endure being put on hold by these misnamed "help" lines for as long as eight hours gave up, and their reimbursement by Plan D for prescription drug costs was sometimes delayed for months. Patients went without critical, life-saving medications for a scandalously long period of time.

Legislation to straighten out this mess and confusion and provide universal health insurance has been blocked for two decades by Big Pharm's and also insurance companies' powerful lobbies and also by hospitals that prefer private insurance because it reimburses them at a higher rate than any proposed by proponents of coverage for all Americans. The current system is complicated beyond intelligibility and unfair to most Americans, riddled with profiteering both legal and illegal. Healthcare at present is a vicious circle; it's like a balloon inflated by problems that will inevitably burst if reforms are not implemented as soon as possible.

The British Bogeyman

Every time health care reform legislation is considered at both the Federal and state level, insurance lobbyists and the Congressmen lodged in their pockets bring up the stalking horse or bogeyman of the National Health Insurance in the U.K., which provides every citizen with coverage, bad-mouthing it as a failed system to discourage the implementation of a similar plan in this country. Their criticism is not only bogus, it is based on the U.K.'s National Health Insurance program of 50 years ago.

When I lived in England from 1969 to 1971 and worked for the National Health Insurance, and then spent the next 36 years in private practice in the U.S., I can say based on my experience with both the U.S. and U.K. systems that the patients in England were treated better than the uninsured or the indigent who are covered by Medicaid in America.

Of course, treatment provided by the National Health Insurance and the hospitals' physical condition was inferior to that of patients with private policies here. Every citizen in the U.K. registers with a general practitioner or primary care physician, who is responsible for providing preventive medical care. Patients with medical problems outside his sphere of the GP's expertise can only be referred to a specialist or even hospital emergency rooms with the permission of their primary care physician.

On the plus side, general practitioners are willing to make house calls for severely ill patients in the U.K., a quaint practice that disappeared in America during the 1950s if not earlier. Plus GPs are not stingy when it comes to sending patients to specialists or emergency rooms.

In 1970, my wife miscarried and suffered mild bleeding. Our general practitioner saw her at home around 9 p.m. and after an examination told my wife that if her condition didn't improve by the following morning, he would refer her to the hospital. If she got worse during the night, he promised to admit her earlier and offered an ambulance to take her to the hospital if the situation became urgent. She did get worse around 2 a.m., we called our GP, and he immediately approved an ambulance, which transported her to the hospital, where she received appropriate treatment.

In the U.K., patients with acute problems will be sent to the ER immediately with no bureaucratic paperwork or delays. But American critics of the U.K.'s socialized medicine accurately point out that for elective surgery, such as operations for hernias, which can linger for a decade without requiring surgical intervention, as well as the removal of benign or nonmalignant tumors, patients are put on a waiting list that can delay their treatment for months. For non-life-threatening problems, doctors prefer to wait until their schedules clear and it's convenient for them to operate.

Another inferior element of medical care in the U.K. compared to the U.S. is the privacy offered by most hospitals in the latter country. In the U.K., public hospitals have something called the "ward system," where 20 patients are crammed into a single ward and few private rooms are available.

But in the last 25 years, the U.K. health system has improved to the point where it approximates the convenience and relative luxury of its American counterparts. Rich Brits now buy additional private insurance so they can check into private hospitals that offer individual rooms that are so luxe that amenities include butler service and gourmet meals, which compared to American hospital food makes tasteless airline dinners seem like Michelin-rated restaurant fare. Private hospitals can afford these posh perks because private insurers in the U.K. reimburse providers handsomely in addition to the national health coverage's payments.

I recently visited a relative in England who was staying at Humana, a private hospital in London. I was impressed with the place, which was the equivalent of or even superior to private hospitals in the U.S. Many private insurers in America refuse to pay for rehab therapy and home healthcare, but the U.K.'s National Health Insurance picks up the tab for both.

The Solution: Medicare for All

The solution to the healthcare crisis involves extending Medicare coverage to every single American, regardless of socio-economic status, including the very rich, and regardless of age. From birth to death or as the British call it, "from cradle to grave."

Presently, Medicare only covers seniors over 65 and the permanently disabled, but reimburses healthcare providers only 80 percent of their allowed costs, while the Medicare recipient must pay the 20 percent balance. Well-off seniors compensate for this by purchasing supplemental private insurance from e.g., Blue Cross/Blue Shield, which pays the 20 percent of allowed charges which Medicare will not.

For the poor and even the middle class, if they were covered by Medicare, the 20 percent out-of-pocket cost for a catastrophic medical bill like $100,000 would be ruinous. My solution for this untenable situation is for the Federal government to allocate funds to build "Medicare hospitals" equivalent to Veterans' Administration hospitals and clinics that exist in every major city. These Medicare-administered hospitals would provide complete service by full-time physicians who are salaried or by part-time physicians on partial salaries.

Today, vets pay nothing at VA hospitals, which typically treat all veterans with or without private insurance or Medicare. Although they are provided medical treatment free of charge, this is not an ideal situation because veterans do not get to see the same doctor every time they seek medical services, which does not provide the comfort of continuity of healthcare—the benefit of seeing the same doctor who is already aware of your medical history and your specific needs that the privately insured enjoy with their regular primary care physicians. But all vets at VA hospitals do get all the healthcare and medicines they need at no cost.

Under my plan for Medicare for all, including prescription drug coverage, there may be a small co-payment required of patients to discourage them for abusing the system with frequent, unnecessary treatments. People within the poverty range or people who use Medicare hospitals to avoid any out-of-pocket expenses will not be charged even this nominal co-payment under my plan.

At my proposed Medicare hospitals and outpatient clinics, staff doctors and part-timers should be reasonably and fairly compensated to ensure that the system does not attract mediocre, under qualified quacks the way so many hospitals for the indigent currently do. A handsome salary will attract competent and bright MDs. If you pay a pittance, you get the dregs of the profession. If a quality physician feels he is still not well compensated enough by Medicare hospitals, he can work part-time and supplement his income in private practice. Physicians fresh out of residency programs do not have enough patients anyway, so Medicare hospitals will supplement their income until their private practice begins to flourish and they pay off all their student loans. The genius of this arrangement is that you get the best doctors who just happen to be newly minted ones.

My Medicare plan will dramatically improve the medical treatment of the poor who can be insured without any out-of-pocket expenses by going to Medicare hospitals. The middle class can choose Medicare hospitals or opt for private hospitals and private physicians if they're willing to pay the 20 percent balance the proposed Medicare plan will not cover if they resist the option of going to *relatively* inferior Medicare hospitals—inferior not in quality of care but lacking the comfort and reassurance of being treated by their personal physician. The middle class will not be negatively impacted by my Medicare plan because some of them will be willing and able to afford the 20 percent co-pay.

The uppermost segment on the socio-economic ladder will probably stick to their current choice of paying for private insurance and private hospitals, while purchasing supplemental insurance to cover my Medicare plan's 20 percent co-pay for hospitalization, doctor office visits and pre-scription medications. The wealthy may also choose to buy deluxe types of insurance that pay healthcare providers more than the current Medicare system does—in return for deluxe medical services.

My Medicare proposal will have to increase doctors' fees in order to off-set the loss of well-to-do privately insured patients who will opt out of my plan. Increased compensation for doctors will encourage the medical com-munity to support a universal Medicare system and also garner the backing of Congressmen who currently balk at the idea of universal healthcare because of the influence of the insurance lobby.

To date, the American Medical Association, another powerful lobby, has blocked any form of health insurance reform. In 1993, the AMA, in addition to hospital groups, insurance companies and prescription drug manufacturers, lobbied to block Hillary Clinton's proposal for universal coverage because doctors feared they would be paid less under her plan. So by raising doctors' and providers' fees with my Medicare plan, there will be less resistance from the AMA. Health insurers were terrified to the point of paranoia that Hillary would put them out of business. My Medicare plan will decrease the revenues of private insurers, but not put them out of business because the well-off will continue to purchase private supplemental insurance instead of relying primarily on private insurance as they do today.

Medical malpractice lawsuit rewards must also be capped to limit Medicare expenses. Currently, patients cannot sue VA hospitals or their staff physicians for malpractice, a rule I would like to see reformed on a national level for all healthcare providers—hospitals and doctors alike.

The proposed Medicare hospitals should be operated with an emphasis on a high level of medical treatment through discipline, oversight and accountability for inferior service. This will encourage patients to access care at Medicare hospitals, making them content and proud, not ashamed as some indigent patients at charity hospitals are now because they feel like second-class citizens, which sadly they are.

The nightmare of shoddy government hospitals was most recently dramatized by the scandal at the Walter Reed Medical Center, a Washington, D.C., VA hospital infested with rats and plagued with crumbling, leaky rooms. The physician in charge of Walter Reed, Major General George W. Weightman, was fired for incompetence even though he had only been on the job for six months and shared limited culpability. The Secretary of the Army, Francis J. Harvey, resigned in disgrace, and the Pentagon was apparently so traumatized by the revelations of mistreatment of Iraq war veterans that it unsuccessfully tried to shutter the entire facility. Accountability and oversight will avoid future scandals like the Walter Reed imbroglio.

Teaching hospitals, which train interns and residents, should also be available to the those who only receive universal Medicare so that everyone will have access to state-of-the-art medicine practiced at university hospitals, including privately insured patients.

To avoid the burdensome paperwork the current Medicare and Medicaid systems generate, the proposed Medicare administration should issue every American a healthcare I.D., which looks like a credit card with his or her picture on it. So when any patient seeks service at a hospital, doctor's office or pharmacy, all he has to do is present his card, have a an electronic print made of it—the equivalent of presenting one's credit card when checking into a hotel. The charges incurred by the Medicare beneficiary will go instantly to Medicare and within two weeks the doctor or pharmacy will receive reimbursement without having to fill out reams of paperwork which create the expense of additional employees to handle it. Most doctors' offices have an employee whose sole duty is to fill out Medicare forms.

At private hospitals, enrollees in the proposed Medicare system should be given an itemized list of the charges for services provided rather than the current mystifying system of simply handing the patient an account of the total cost of services, which allows some hospital to commit fraud by overcharging Medicare. An itemized list will allow the patient to determine if the hospital has charged for services not performed.

(Private health insurers already provide itemized lists. A friend of mine recently received a claim form from a doctor he had never seen or even heard of, billing almost $3,000 for such procedures as a pap smear and medical equipment only used by females, even though my friend is a male!)

The new Medicare non-profit hospitals will not be tempted to over bill or commit fraud for unnecessary services because all their doctors will be salaried, not reimbursed per service. Salaried physicians will also result in a simplification of the billing process and reduce overheard for doctors and hospitals. When visiting private hospitals or private physicians, patients have to present their Medicare card and sign for any services rendered. They should be given an itemized statement listing the charges for treatment. They need to check the statement before they sign it and leave in the same way that they do when people check out of hotels. The charges will be transferred immediately to Medicare electronically, and the provider will be reimbursed within two weeks.

Medicare for All Will Reduce Prescription Drug Costs

As a single agent, the new Medicare system will negotiate with drug companies on behalf of a whopping constituency with the clout of 300 million

Americans. Medicare can choose one or two brands of drugs per disease that act in identical fashion, and drugs companies will find themselves losing their share of the market if they don't agree to Medicare's demands to slash their prices. The Canadian government has already used its leverage to force American drug companies to offer deep discounts, which has created the caravans of Americans who cross the border to fill their prescriptions at Canadian pharmacies. Even though this is illegal, that hasn't stopped seniors terrified of having a heart attack or stroke because they can't afford American-priced drugs for hypertension. Fear of death trumps fear of Federal prison.

Under my plan, drug manufacturers will be dealing with only one agent, Medicare, which will be able to negotiate huge discounts and prices only slightly above the cost of production, still providing the drug makers with a fair profit—rather than their current obscene profits because they now charge six times what it costs them to produce medications. Drug companies will be forced to cooperate; if they don't, Medicare will inform them that it will no longer do business with them. Holding a monopoly on drug purchases, Medicare will not allow drug manufacturers an alternative market where they can gouge pharmacies and patients.

The system, however, will not eliminate consumer choice. If the patient wants a specific brand name drug not on Medicare's formulary—a list of drugs Medicare agrees to reimburse for—the patient can pay for his preferred drug out of pocket.

The new Medicare administration will have to be on guard to stop government bureaucrats from accepting kickbacks from drug companies in return for accepting higher prescription medication prices. Such as the Halliburton Company, formerly headed by Vice President Cheney receiving overpriced contracts from the U.S. government for services provided in Iraq. Medicine should be provided with a low-cost co-payment at Medicare hospitals and clinics to avoid abuse.

Critics, especially Republicans who claim less government is more, will object to Medicare's further Federal intrusion into the lives of American citizens (although they never object when government "intrudes" in abortion and gay rights issues), but if the new system is managed fairly and efficiently, the uninsured and indigent Medicaid beneficiaries, which together currently comprise a shameful one third of the population, will fare much better than the current system.

The current Medicare Plan D, which provides ultra low prescription drug prices for seniors and the disabled often with nominal or no co-pays and deductibles, uses approximately 20 different insurance company plans in each state and negotiates separate deals and prices with drug manufacturers. This dilution of Plan D's clout allows drug companies to, say, lose five to ten bids and still have a chance at winning ten others. The negotiating power of drug makers will be exponentially reduced because under the new system there will be only one "insurance plan," i.e. Medicare, to negotiate with, not 20 different plans per state.

The new Medicare should appoint a panel of knowledgeable, specialist physicians, with no ties to any drug company to set a fair price for prescription medications and offer drug companies a take-it-or-leave-it choice on whether to accept the set prices. Medicare will be able to reject any drug for its beneficiaries if the drug makers don't fall in line as well as reward drug suppliers who do accept the mandated price.

All of the above recommendations will eliminate the consternation of the population which falls outside Medicare's current coverage limited to seniors over 65 and the disabled who can't afford private insurance, those who depend on the whims of bean-counting employers who eliminate employee insurance coverage at the first whiff of rising premiums, and those who resent managed care plans that tell them which doctors they can see and which hospitals they can go to. Employees will not fear the loss of their health insurance through layoffs or terminations because Medicare will guarantee continued coverage regardless of their employment status.

If we accept universal health coverage with open and generous minds, the new system may not be the best of all possible worlds, but infinitely better than the current system with its massive uninsured portions of the population, which is the worst of all possible worlds. With time, Medicare will evolve based on experience, enabling it to make changes that improve services.

To Recap

It is the inalienable right of every American citizen to have basic healthcare coverage paid for by the United States government. It's our nation's basic duty that is already fulfilled by all other industrialized nations. Western Europe, Japan, Canada and Australia take care of their citizens' healthcare needs, and it's past due that the richest of these industrialized nations follows their lead.

If well-off Americans find the new Medicare system does not meet their needs, they can pay out of pocket for supplemental insurance the way many affluent seniors over 65 on Medicare do today. This supplemental insurance premium will be a bargain compared to primary private insurers' premiums at present because the new Medicare will pay 80 percent of every American's—rich or poor—insurance costs, while the well-heeled will only have to shell out the remaining 20 percent for private supplemental insurance.

Although it may seem heartless, we have to set a limit on how long and how extensively we can continue to treat terminally ill or hopeless cases that drain huge amounts from a finite pool of funds so that this money can be spent on salvageable lives and benefit the majority of the population rather than the minority of hopeless cases. It's a Hobbesian choice, but one that must be made.

Providers—physicians and hospitals—may object to expanding Medicare to cover all Americans because they fear losing the higher reimbursements currently offered by private insurers. But these naysayers must be reminded that the new Medicare plan will cover the lower third income group—the uninsured and the indigent on Medicaid—the same group providers complain stress their resources because Medicaid reimburses them with shamefully small amounts and the uninsured often simply default on their doctor and hospital debts.

Providers may be paid less by Medicare than by current private insurers, but those who can afford private insurance will probably buy supplemental coverage under the new system and this insurance will make up for what doctors and hospitals lose when private insurers are dissolved.

Who's Gonna Pay For All This?

At present, every employed American pays 1.45 percent of his gross income to support the Medicare fund. The monthly payroll deduction ranges from $80 to $120 depending on the taxpayer's income. These taxpayers won't be able to access Medicare until they turn 65, when they are likely to have more health-related problems than during their prime working years during which they are relatively healthier and don't need as much medical care as seniors do.

Many Americans under 65 also have private insurance, which employers may or may not subsidize. The average employee pays between $300 and $360 per month for individual coverage, depending on age and past illnesses. If the employee's dependents are also covered by his private insurance, this additional coverage can add $600 to $700 per month or an average 25 percent of his gross income. Many middle-class employees find that paying close to $1,000 per month for private insurance takes too big a bite out of their paycheck, and they often drop coverage, further enlarging the rolls of the uninsured, whose numbers, as already noted, are growing at an average of five million every two to five years.

So the middle class currently pays for healthcare at the rate of 13 to 15 percent of his gross income in the form of Medicare taxes and the premiums on individual private insurance. Adding dependents can increase premiums to 25 percent of gross income (an average salary of $3,000 per month for an employee with an annual income of $36,000).

My reform of Medicare will cover all Americans from cradle to grave. The increased cost for this extended coverage will be paid for by increasing the Medicare tax from the current rate of 1.45 percent to 5 to 8 percent. with the higher percentage paid by employees with dependents. I can already hear Republicans howling: "Read my lips. Americans don't want new taxes!" But in fact, they may already pay double the equivalent of the proposed increase in Medicare taxes—5 to 8 percent—in the form of private insurance premiums, deductibles, copayments, prescription drugs, etc.

But this additional tax, instead of going toward "unsexy" things like improving infrastructure (Americans would presumably prefer to drive over potholes rather than open their wallets for more taxes) or developing alternative fuel sources (poisonous air rather than less money to spend at Wal-Mart), will directly impact employees by providing them with afford-able healthcare, which polls show is one of the most pressing concerns of the American public and the same polls indicate that voters are willing to pay more to avoid the nightmare of getting catastrophically sick with no insurance to protect them. And for decades, Americans have been com-plaining about the ever-increasing expense and unavailability of private insurance, especially for the self-employed, the unemployed and those on limited incomes.

Employees can also be made more amenable to paying higher taxes for Medicare coverage by the government requiring their employers to raise their wages 10 percent and increase the minimum wage to $10 an hour, which will offset employees' increased outlay for Medicare. Now, before employers start howling about raising wages, they will also be mollified by the realization that when their employees are covered by Medicare, they won't have to subsidize the ever-rising premiums they pay for their work-ers' private health insurance. In short, employers will pay higher salaries but enjoy huge savings by not paying for private coverage. And workers will enjoy increased wages to pay for the increase in Medicare taxes.

Everyone will be happy except the insurance lobby, whose corrupt influence on lawmakers, as described in Chapter One, will be eroded by the creation of a third, independent party that allied with liberal Demo-crats will make an end-run around the insurance lobby and crush their unconscionable practices once and for all. For the new Medicare system to be accepted and not blocked by physician, hospital and drug manufacturer lobbies, providers must be made happy and content with fair and decent compensation, which my plan will provide for all but the greediest of pro-viders. The maddening hegemony of the insurance lobby will wither and die.

The administrative costs of Medicare at present (paperwork, extra employees, etc.) is approximately three percent, an impressive and tiny amount of the total cost of the program compared to the wasteful (or even fraudulent) administrative costs of private insurance and managed care

(HMOs), which range from 15 to 20 percent, according to a 2007 interview with Hillary Clinton, whose plan for universal health coverage in 1993 went down in flames and recriminations during her husband's administration.

The excess profits of private insurance companies can be confiscated and transferred to the Medicare pot so beneficiaries will enjoy even broader health care coverage. Universal healthcare will improve the quality of life of lower income Americans who are uninsured and the indigent who suffer under the parsimonious Medicaid program, which is inferior to Medicare coverage.

Not just the working poor and indigent will benefit from my Medicare plan. The middle class, which is struggling with ruinous deductibles, mediocre coverage, and arbitrary, huge and yearly raises in their premiums, will also be big winners under my plan. They will make co-payments for their prescription drugs as members of HMOs do now.

If Medicare coverage isn't sumptuous enough for the wealthy, they can afford supplemental private insurance which will keep their healthcare providers happy with higher reimbursements.

With the expansion of Medicare, we will have one universal system, no confusion, and an equitable distribution of the cost of healthcare. Universal healthcare will be fair and end the current universal resentment of price-gouging by providers.

In his 2007 book, *Sick: The Untold Story of America's Health Care Crisis—And the People Who Pay the Price*, Jonathan Cohn reports that currently the United States pays approximately 16 percent of its gross domestic product on healthcare, but the quality of the nation's healthcare ranks far below that of other industrialized nations'. The United Kingdom pays only seven percent of its GDP for healthcare, which may be only of average quality, with necrotic hospitals and clinics 100 years or older.

But France provides a happier example of government-sponsored healthcare, which is usually rated No. 1 in surveys, while the nation spends much less than the U.S. but more than the United Kingdom does providing adequate medical treatment, and its citizens have easy access to the system. One of the ways France achieves excellence on the cheap is by controlling the use of high tech medicines and state-of-the-art medical procedures so they can't be employed indiscriminately if there is no proof of their efficacy and a good clinical outcome. Many desperate cancer patients in America demand bone marrow transplants even though studies have shown they prolong life minimally if at all. France deals with this scientific fact simply by refusing to pay for such transplants.

Even in its current, less than perfect incarnation, Medicare is simple and runs smoothly, with low administrative costs. With Medicare, patients can see any doctor they want or check into the hospital of their choice. Unlike private insurers, Medicare doesn't refuse to pay for pre-existing conditions and also unlike many private insurers it reimburses for mental healthcare, physical therapy and chiropractic.

Medicare is not flawless. It still needs to better compensate providers—physicians, hospitals, dialysis and outpatient clinics—because Medicare's current rate of reimbursement has not kept up with the rising cost of living over the past 30 years. Doctors should be reimbursed equitably, based on the length of their training. (Plastic surgeons, for example, do an eight rather than four-year residency in part because they are required to take exotic courses in sculpture and facial aesthetics.)

Specialists should all receive the same pay, unlike the current Medicare system in which anesthesiologists and orthopedic surgeons are paid inexplicably much more than other specialists, while pediatricians, internists and psychiatrists are the least compensated.

CHAPTER SIX
Saving Our Children's Education

One of the most important measures of a nation's greatness is its ability to provide every one of its children a quality education. By this standard of national excellence, America is failing catastrophically. And there's no good reason for this failure. Although the United States has more Nobel Laureates than any other country in the world, as well as more doctors, attorneys, engineers and military personnel, it is also tragically home to 21 million illiterate adults, according to a report by the National Jewish Coalition for Literacy in 2007. Another study the same year by another research group reported that *40* million adults in the U.S. are illiterate.

This group of truly lost souls in an increasingly sophisticated economy that requires increasingly well-trained workers constitutes 25 percent of the adult population. This is a staggering percentage of illiteracy compared to other industrialized nations in Europe as well as Canada, Australia, Japan and South Korea, among others.

The effects of illiteracy go beyond creating a pool of unemployable workers. According to the National Jewish Coalition, 70 percent of Americans arrested are illiterate, 85 percent of unwed mothers are illiterate, and one in five high school graduates cannot read his or her diploma. The coalition estimates that illiteracy costs the United States $225 billion a year in lost productivity.

This legion of the damned cannot decipher any text or comprehend what they read. Solving simple math problems that an average third grader can easily accomplish mystifies these unfortunates. They are condemned to no-status, dead-end, minimum-wage jobs because they cannot fill out a simple job application—forget about creating an eye-catching résumé—or interpret the instructional manuals for operating machinery.

Although millions of these illiterates are high school graduates, they know nothing about academics and far too much about athletics, which seems to be the main focus of their so-called education in grades K through 12. They may be brilliant athletes but possess the reading skills of a third grader, which is no skill at all. They understand goal lines but not academic goals.

I once asked a co-worker, a nurse, if her son's school was any good, and her reply was, "Yes, they have an excellent football team." Unfortunately, too many Americans measure the quality of their schools, including colleges, by their achievements in athletics, not academics. This phenomenon is more prevalent in public than in private schools. The parents of children in private schools pay exorbitant tuition and are motivated to get their money's worth so they care more about their kids' scholarly progress than their ability to kick a field goal.

If these affluent parents were more interested in sports than academics, they wouldn't waste their resources on pricy private academies. If their goal were turning their child into the best jock he or she can possibly be, the public school system would do quite nicely, thank you. Students contribute to the problem because they have a natural tendency to favor sports, which are fun, not math and science, which often seem recondite and irrelevant.

A friend of mine, a nationally known political columnist, fretted about her high-school aged daughter flunking calculus and the effect it would have on her college admissions prospects, so she hired a tutor and as soon as the girl's calculus grade rose to a C, she terminated the private instructor in the belief that calculus would have no relevance to her life and career as an adult.

Most Americans are frustrated by the poor level of education offered by public schools, more so in the South than in the Northeast, Midwest or West. I live in Chattanooga, Tennessee, and many of my friends feel compelled to send their children to private schools for a more academically-oriented education, often at great economic hardship—the average annual tuition at a top college-prep academy is $30,000—because they see no alternative to the pom-pom and football jersey form of what passes as learning at too many public schools.

During every presidential and mid-term election, politicians pay lip service decrying the scandalous state of public education, but as soon as they win, their concerns evaporate. The current administration and legislative branches have been particularly guilty of not—so-benign neglect. Education reform is not a priority for them. But it will have to become a priority if Republicans expect to make a credible showing in the 2008 election.

In 2006, *Education Week* magazine reported that an impressive majority, 62 percent, of those polled believed that Democrats care more about education reform than Republicans, whom only a small minority, 17 percent, felt would do a better job at educating our youth. These statistics may explain in part the 2006 loss of both the House and the Senate by the Republicans, and why Democratic candidates in general fare better in polls for the 2008 race.

The public preference for Democrats over Republicans when it comes to education is more likely due to talk rather than action. Both parties have been remiss in addressing the myriad of problems confronting public education, but in debates the Democrats at least talk about it more than their Republican rivals.

During a debate among Republican presidential hopefuls in Los Angeles in May 2007, the candidates obsessed about abortion and gay rights while failing to even bring up the issues Americans care much more about, like affordable health insurance, education and crime reform.

As noted in earlier chapters, it is the duty of every nation to provide a free and high quality education for all its children—as important as affordable healthcare, crime reduction, air that doesn't make your eyes water or water that tastes like rotten eggs, and strong national security against domestic terrorism. Many believe that throwing money at the problem, pumping more funds into the educational pool, will solve the problem, but this is a fallacy.

More money for schools is an important factor for improving them, but it is only one of many. Before we try to raise educational standards, we have to find the reasons the current system produces 21 million people—25 percent of the adult population—who can't decipher the headlines in their daily newspapers reporting the latest massacre of Iraqi civilians or President Bush's giveaway tax cuts for billionaires.

An illiterate electorate may partially explain the continued legislative inaction on ending the war in Iraq. If you can't *read* newspaper reports that 1,000 Americans soldiers are dying every year in Iraq, you can't *write* your Congressman or Senators demanding they stop the bloodshed.

Our Broken Educational System and How to Fix It

Problem No. 1: Children are not indoctrinated during their learning years about why they are legally required to attend school at least until age 16. Are their goals academic, athletic or social? They need to be told what their priorities must be. This is the job of parents, who need to "brain wash" their children through repeated lectures that the primary reason for school attendance is academic excellence, not how to hit the basket from the free-throw line or wear cool clothes to class.

College should be presented to students as the Holy Grail of education primarily so they will get a good, professional job after graduation, although personal enrichment and exposure to new ideas are equally valid reasons for higher education—they just don't translate into handsome paychecks. High school football stars with dreams of pro gridiron glory should be reminded of the sad statistic that only a tiny percentage of college football players make it to the pros. Ditto for basketball, baseball, wrestling and golf jocks, etc.

If parents can't afford to pay their children's' college tuition, that is no excuse to skip the educational opportunity of a lifetime. There are always scholarships, grants and government-guaranteed loans (although the present administration has tried to cut back such loans to their great shame) that will help them navigate the financial shoals of higher education.

If a student simply doesn't have the "smarts"—low grade-point averages, shabby SAT scores—they still need not be condemned to the life of minimum-wage helots, degreasing French fries at Burger King. Vocational or trade schools are a great alternative, and graduates with much valued technical skills to become plumbers, electricians and IT experts often earn as much if not more than graduates of traditional four-year colleges. And they can be out of vocational school in only two!

Parental influence and guidance are imperative because students' peers will fill the vacuum left by apathetic parents by encouraging them to drop out of high school, join gangs, experiment with drugs and commit crime. Parents must oversee their children's education all the way from K through 12th grades. Unfortunately, too many adults are so preoccupied working long hours to keep up with the middle class's declining earning power that they don't have the time or energy to monitor their children's academic progress, or lack thereof.

Some are so indifferent to the inferior quality of their children's schools they don't start complaining until report cards turn up pockmarked with Ds and Fs. At home, parents should play the role of school counselors while teachers encourage their charges during school hours. Twelve years of education should be a form of programming to achieve academic excellence and admission to college or vocational schools.

No. 2: The emphasis on sports achievement at the expense of academic accomplishment is a nationwide disgrace. Although sports are important for building character, teaching cooperation for the common good, reversing the current epidemic of childhood obesity, yah-de-yah-de-yah-de, athletics should rate a distant second to scholastics. Parents often brag about their son's prowess on the football field or their daughter's soccer goals, but they need to praise them even more fulsomely when they come home with a report card festooned with As or make the Dean's List.

Understandably, parents on a budget whose children are mediocre students often encourage them to excel at sports in the hope of landing an athletic scholarship because they can't afford the stiff tuition fees of higher education. I personally know many parents who let their children devote all their after-class time to athletics at the expense of studying. These kids are so occupied with sports, I wonder when they have time to do their homework. Probably, many simply don't, hence the D and F report cards.

Colleges are also culprits in sports-crazy America. They offer more athletic than academic scholarships, a bass-ackward practice since they're called institutions of higher *learning*, not higher basketball scores. Worse, recipients of athletic "scholarships"—a misnomer if ever there was one—tend to be C and D students, and their inferior educational skills drag down the entire student body and diminish scholastic morale because college athletes are treated like heroes. They, and not intellectual geeks, tend to be unacceptable role models.

No. 3: Lack of discipline. Students often cannot be punished or expelled if they engage in disruptive behavior because of various laws that protect students rights. In many states, spanking is forbidden by statute, and you can't infringe on students' freedom, which often translates as the right to goof off.

When I was in the equivalent of grade and high school in Egypt, if someone misbehaved, he was punished outside the classroom. We were motivated to behave because we knew justice would be swift and severe in the form of spanking. For extra humiliation and deterrence, corporal punishment sometimes took place in front of the class. Serious misbehavior elicited even harsher retribution—expulsion for a day or forever.

Today, in America, too often the teacher is "wrong," and the student is "right." That is the prevailing attitude in public schools especially. In earlier times and even now in other countries, the opposite was true. The lack of discipline is often mandated by parents, who are the first to object to school punishment. Parents lack the will or involvement to discipline their children at home, and they don't want anyone to usurp their parental obligations at school.

As a result, children grow up misguided, contemptuous of authority and rules, disruptive and even violent. Their bad example influences otherwise good students to follow their path to dropping out and hanging out or holding down coolie-wage, dead-end jobs.

No. 4: Unqualified, inexperienced and poorly paid teachers. A Princeton University study shows that 67 percent of science and math teachers on the high school level do not have degrees in the subjects they teach. Lack of interest in math and science often begins at the grade school level and extends into college, where graduates choose not to major in those two difficult subjects. More lucrative offers to work in private industry also lure math and science majors away from academe.

The Princeton report said it is very difficult to attract science graduates to the teaching profession, so schools end up hiring teachers who haven't majored in chemistry, math, physics or biology and who are unqualified to teach those subjects. For example, if you had a brain tumor, would you want treatment by a podiatrist?

Another problem contributing to the mediocrity of public school education is that teachers are not required to be recertified at regular intervals, and many states do not require them to pursue continuing education or training on a yearly basis. Teachers must remain at a certain level of excellence to continue their careers. Some testing takes place on the local and state levels, but the tests should be standardized and applied nationwide to make sure that every student in the country is receiving the same level of educational excellence.

Other professions already recognize the need for standardized, national tests. American physicians have to be recertified every 10 years by passing a national examination. They also have to take 20 to 50 hours of continuing education every year in order to maintain a valid license. Teachers should meet the same requirements to keep their knowledge of the latest pedagogical theories and practices up to date.

No. 5: Lack of accountability for poorly performing teachers and schools. Testing students will determine if their teachers and schools are doing a good job. Teachers should be rewarded for good test results achieved by students and eliminated, i.e., fired, for consistently bad test results. Harsh, but the rest of our children's lives are at stake, and they cannot be sacrificed on the altar of incompetent instructors and disengaged school districts.

On the state level, school superintendents or supervisors must take a hands-on approach, visit classes, monitor the teachers' lecturing acumen and question students to determine their level of achievement on every academic subject—English, math, physical and social sciences, civics, American history and at least one foreign language.

No. 6: No minimum academic curriculum. In my home state of Tennessee, math instruction is very primitive, and there is no requirement to learn a second language, even though Spanish is quickly becoming the nation's second tongue as the population of immigrants from Latin America continues to balloon, and Latinos have surpassed blacks as the largest minority group in the country according to the 2000 Census.

Too many schools allow students to design their own curriculum, and they tend to take the easy route and enroll in undemanding classes like art, interior design, home ec, and pseudo-social science courses such as "sports theory."

The urgency of improving math education in particular is underlined by the current phenomenon that when students finish high school, they test at the 7th or 8th grade level of math. High school seniors are unable to solve simple arithmetic problems that in later life will be required for such everyday tasks as balancing a checkbook, figuring out the monthly payments on their mortgage or determining what, say, a 50 percent markdown on clothing amounts to. We're not talking about the mystifying universe of calculus here.

There are no mandatory make-up classes for those falling behind in math; instead students gravitate to non-challenging "subjects" like sports, drawing, culinary arts, fashion merchandising—all of which would be better taught at vocational schools.

Minimum academic requirements should be the equivalent or superior of other industrialized nations' standards. The length of the school day should also be increased, lasting from 8 a.m. to 4 p.m., with all athletic activities beginning no earlier than 2 p.m.

If we want to remain the world's only superpower with the ability to thwart ethnic cleansing and other atrocities committed by much less powerful nations, science education must also be improved, and yet only an anemic 37 percent of respondents to an *Education Week* poll "strongly agree" that "science education in U.S. schools is poor to mediocre. Thirty-seven percent is a start, but until more parents demand that science courses rise above the current poor to mediocre rating, we will fall behind as a benevolent superpower as we crank out less and less scientists who we need to make sure we remain the strongest superpower as well.

It is time to be firm and not worry about such feel-good goals as maintaining our children's self-esteem by insisting that high school students meet minimum requirements in math and science or they don't graduate. Creating more college-prep courses in those subjects will help students pass standardized national tests.

No. 7: No testing of students on a yearly basis. On the state level, testing should be conducted annually. On the national level, tests might be administered at the sixth, ninth and twelfth grades. Each state's testing results should be compared to the national standard, and each school should compare its performance to its state's standard.

Southern states suffer the lowest test scores of any region in the country. If these states required annual testing, they would know the level of their educational performance compared to other states, the South would be required to administer the same standardized tests as the rest of the nation.

In a practice euphemistically known as "social promotion," students automatically progress to the next grade regardless of their academic performance during the past year, even if they are failing the class. This may seem like a kind way of not holding back or embarrassing low-performing students, but this perceived kindness actually does them a disservice because they end up earning high school diplomas which some of them can't even read, leaving them woefully unqualified for all but the most menial of jobs.

In other countries not all students are promoted to the next grade (10 to 20 percent are held back on average), an effective motivation to ensure that everyone studies hard and avoids the public humiliation of repeating the grade.

In a January 2001 report by the Southern Regional Education Board in Atlanta, the organization explained exactly why bumping unqualified students up to the next grade harms rather than comforts them: "Social promotion is unfair to students and detrimental to society. These students typically fall further and further behind their classmates."

And many don't even have the minor blessing of leaving school with a diploma, however unindicative the sheepskin is of their achievements, because these students "ultimately leave school without the basic skills and knowledge every adult needs to be a productive member of society," according to the Atlanta educational board.

Although mandatory retention has been going on for decades, the Atlanta board says research shows it does not work, and the frustrated student often leaves before graduating: "The preponderance of evidence on retention strongly indicates that retention rarely does much good and often can do considerable harm. The research is particularly clear on one significant point: being required to repeat even one grade ... dramatically increases the likelihood that a student will drop out of school. Few students who repeat more than one grade will complete high school."

This harmful practice is also widespread. The board reported that 15 to 20 percent of all students repeat at least one grade between the ages of six and seventeen. Seven million students will be retained at least once. And the burden falls most heavily on society's most disadvantaged: "Poor and minority students are two to three times more likely than others to be retained."

The Atlanta board recommended that instead of waiting until the conclusion of the school year to determine if the student has failed, early intervention *during* the school term will help identify struggling students and give them "extra time" to catch up and provide tutors, with each remedial program specifically designed to each troubled student's needs rather than the unworkable cookie-cutter approach of mandatory retention.

The board's report concluded: "Providing struggling students with the right kinds and amounts of extra help during the school year is more complicated and demanding than promoting or retaining these students, but it is the only way to avoid dooming millions of children to continued failure. It may be the only way to make education

reform and accountability work."

No. 8: Parental participation. The schools aren't the only group responsible for guaranteeing academic achievement. Parents must get involved as much as teachers. At least from the first through sixth grades, if not earlier, parents should tutor their children in the home to supplement what they learn in the classroom. Past sixth grade, parents may not be qualified academically to continue their tutorship, but they should still monitor and guide their children, charting their progress in school to make sure they are not falling behind.

To date, parents don't seem to be getting this message of the need for more involvement in their children's education. Only 39 percent of parents polled by *Education Week* "agree" that "most high school students are not motivated to do their best." Before the school day even begins, parents should give their kids a kind but firm lecture on how important the rest of the day will be to their future, especially their careers, and instill in them a sense of discipline, which need not consist of anything more complicated than "pay attention to what the teacher is telling you" and "don't be disruptive" so the other children will also have a shot at learning.

To maximize their own learning potential, children must be protected against severely disruptive students, who bring guns, alcohol or drugs on campus. If these activities plague your school, contact the principal and demand that action be taken against these delinquents. If the situation doesn't improve, make hell at the school-superintendent level or with your city's elected officials.

Teachers are remiss in not assigning students more homework, and children waste their after-school hours playing mind-obliterating video games, watching TV and trawling the Internet. Private schools tend to require more homework, one of the many reasons that account for their superior academic record. I recommend public schools mandate a minimum of three hours per night.

No. 9: One cause of substandard education: Excessive funds are wasted bussing students to and from school. Sometimes parents are able to drive their children, but too many of them opt for the convenience and savings—financial and time—by letting schools take responsibility for their children's transportation. With more parents willing to carpool, funds previously spent on bussing could be used to pay for other school programs, renovation of school facilities and grounds, a fresh coat of paint so students don't feel like they're attending a bombed-out building in post-war Berlin, and more computers and science lab equipment.

This recommendation is not heartless or all-encompassing. Bussing should be provided free of charge for indigent students and others living in remote areas where the cost of transportation may be prohibitively expensive even for middle-class parents. If well-off parents still resist the inconvenience of *schlepping* their kids to school, they should be required to pay for transportation, as many private schools already do.

Bussing to achieve racial parity should be ended—period. Even minority students loathe bussing because it requires so much extra time traveling to distant schools. Bussing to improve education is also unnecessary because the curriculum at all schools, regardless of their location, should be improved and educational parity, rather than racial parity, achieved in that manner. The money saved from needless bussing can be spent on improving infrastructure and academic programs.

No. 10: Not enough vocational or technical training. Let's be upfront and not squeamish. Some students, for many reasons which are and aren't their fault, are simply not college material, and the last two years of high school are wasted on academic courses which a: they may fail and b: bear no practical relevance to their post-school careers. Junior and senior years for the bottom 25 percent of students, who have no plans of going on to college, should be devoted to learning a trade to become plumbers, electricians, carpenters, bricklayers, computer repairmen and auto mechanics.

After graduation, they can spend an additional year as interns, gaining practical, on-the-job experience. Vocational schools and internships will provide them with well-paying jobs with the extra bonus of earning a high school diploma that spares them from the minimum-wage slave status that currently awaits them after dropping out or being "socially promoted" to cap and gown.

No. 11: Not enough magnet schools. These institutions are called "magnets" because they offer a sophisticated curriculum which, like magnets, attract the top 25 percent of students with courses on classical Greek and Latin, algebra II, performing arts, painting, sculpting, obscure foreign languages, advanced computer skills—a cornucopia of academic riches for children who want to get the very best out of their education. At least these magnet schools *should* be attracting the top 25 percent of overachievers.

But in my home state of Tennessee and elsewhere, admission to these coveted schools is on a first-come, first-served basis, with prior academic achievement ignored by the admissions process. Transferring to magnet schools can begin in the sixth or ninth grade. If these students perform poorly, they should be banished to their regular schools and replaced by the next level of top grade-earners who failed to gain admission to magnet schools on their first try.

Magnet schools should also add more AP (advanced placement, college-credit) courses to their curricula to improve their students' chances of gaining admission to top universities. One foreign language should be mandatory and two optional at magnet schools. Public schools should require its students to learn one foreign language as well so as adults they can compete in a global economy.

Unfortunately, less than a majority (41 percent) of parents polled by *Education Week* "strongly agree" and only 25 percent "agree" with me on the need for more "magnetic" subjects and schools. Despite their parents' lack of enthusiasm, their children seem to be extremely attracted by magnet schools because so many of them are turned away for lack of openings.

This will of course mean more money needs to be extracted from parsimonious legislators, but if only 25 percent of public schools were transformed into magnets, there would be enough slots open to accommodate all the students who are currently being turned away at the door.

And this is my response to the 14 percent of parents polled by *Education Week* who "strongly disagree" that more magnet schools are needed: Don't send your kids there. Simple enough.

No. 12: Too many "bad apples" spoiling the rest of the barrel. To avoid distracting students who want to learn, disruptive youngsters should be transferred to separate schools where they can receive the additional counseling they so obviously need and learn a code of ethics and responsibility toward their peers and society in general.

Really bad apples—violent youth who bring guns and drugs to campus—should be expelled because they may be hazardous to the intellectual and physical wellbeing of the rest of the student body. The Columbine and Amish school tragedies could have been averted if the teen shooters had been identified and preemptively removed from their schools.

Solution No. 1: Standardized testing of students. Statewide testing of all students should be conducted on an annual basis. Nationwide testing should take place at grades six, nine and twelve. The tests should focus on college-prep education, such as foreign languages, math, science, history and the humanities—not the "theory" of how sportsmanship builds character and improves self-esteem through athletic participation, just a few of the bogus courses offered by schools.

The No Child Left Behind Act of 2001, which was backed by President Bush and signed into law by him in January 2002 and which, according to the Associated Press, is "vital to Bush's agenda and his legacy," mandates statewide testing of children in reading and math in grades three through eight and once in high school. Schools that receive Federal funding must demonstrate academic progress or face financial sanctions. The law was intended to pressure schools into paying more attention to children who test poorly.

During a speech at the White House in April 2007 in front of supporters of the act, which was up for renewal that year, teachers told the President several times that statewide tests are not effective because state standards are a hodgepodge nationwide and agreed with me that there must also be standardized *nationwide* testing.

A dissident group of parents polled by the Associated Press, 40 percent, complained that schools put too much emphasis on getting kids to pass tests rather than measuring educational achievement by other means, although the dissidents didn't specify an alternative means of measurement. However, 41 percent of parents want nationwide testing.

Parents' perception of the effectiveness of testing tends to depend on their own education. The more highly educated want more, not less, testing. These parents often send their children to excellent private schools, and they are proud of the fact that they score at the top of their class.

The dissidents, who tend to be more poorly educated, are uninformed about the importance of gauging their children's academic progress, and because their children often score at the bottom of the tests they are embarrassed and even paranoid that testing will make their children look bad. These selfish adults don't care if the nation's standard of education improves, including—shockingly—the quality of their own kids' education.

But the uninformed and ill-educated aren't the only opponents of this crucial law. According to a 2003 poll, almost 50 percent of school principals and superintendents view the No Child Left Behind Act as either politically motivated or aimed at undermining public schools. These derelict educators also felt testing was unfair to the poor and minorities, who tend to score poorly. The poll neglected to inquire if these disgruntled educators headed poorly performing schools which they felt were being "undermined"—although "embarrassed" is probably a more likely description of the reason for their vote of no confidence.

Senator Hillary Clinton is also an exception to the generalization that the No Child Left Behind Act is rejected mostly by the uneducated who don't value their children's education. Although a graduate of the ultra elite Seven Sisters' Wellesley College and Yale Law School who voted for the act in 2001, Clinton has apparently since then had a change of heart. In a speech before the New York State United Teachers' annual convention held in Washington, D.C., she blasted the act as putting too much weight on standardized testing and undermining student creativity.

Clinton didn't reject the idea of educational reform, but she felt the act was not providing it. "We can all agree that we do need measures," she told the teachers' convention on April 27, 2007. "We do need accountability. But not the kind of accountability that the NCLB law has imposed on people." Clinton complained that the act has received less funding than originally promised by its proponents. Standardized testing, she insisted, had become a case of the tail wagging the dog: "The tests have become the curriculum instead of the other way around. It's time we had a President who cares more about learning than memorizing." Clinton was preaching to the choir, i.e., the New York State United Teachers union, whose 575,000 members have slammed the act for its punitive nature and inflexibility.

There *is* a place for what Clinton calls "creativity" in education, but it should take the form of optional classes in such artsy-craftsy subjects as, well, arts and crafts, culinary arts, auto repair, drafting and carpentry, cosmetology and the lamentable but inevitable "sports theory," *et al.*

While the academic requirements of the No Child Left Behind Act need to be reauthorized, there is compelling evidence that they also need to be revamped and the level of excellence dramatically raised. The Center on Education Policy, a nonpartisan Washington, D.C.-based advocacy group for more effective public schools, said that after three years of collecting data, 31 states reported that math scores for public elementary school students had improved.

But before you send flowers to your child's third grade teacher or a tax-deductible donation to the non-profit Center on Education Policy, it should be noted that the math scores improved by a breath-taking … one percent! Twenty-nine states reported that a similar percentage of reading scores had also improved, which the Center on Education Policy grandiosely characterized as "moderate to large."

Five states collected enough data to show improvement in math and reading scores in elementary, middle and high schools, but again an increase of only one percent, which one cock-eyed optimist school superintendent crowed was "higher than expected." One wonders what percentage increase the superintendent would call "lower than expected.

The importance of math and science for K through 12th grade students cannot be overstated. Unfortunately, this belief receives only tepid support from parents, with only 43 percent agreeing that "improving math and science instruction should be the top priority for K through 12 schools," according to a poll conducted by *Education Week* in May 2007. If we want to compete on a global level and not outsource our work to Third-World countries like India, our children must master math and science.

Fortunately, the AP poll showed that only five percent "strongly disagree" that we need more, not less, standardized testing on the national level. Probably both they and their children are underachievers who lack motivation and do not care about learning since my guess is that the parents' own educational experience was not a happy one and did not lead to a lucrative job after graduation from high school. These irresponsible adults are pessimists who suspect that their children are incapable of improving their proficiency in math and science.

We have to educate these dissenters about the need to improve their children's education. If we don't, their kids will end up at the bottom of their schools' academic rankings, and their chances at college and the good life will be virtually nil. When we require children to compete via nationwide testing, it motivates them to study harder and pay more attention in class so they score well on tests. When apathetic parents see visual proof of their children's academic improvement, they will change their minds about the importance of regular testing.

No. 2: Standardized testing of teachers and accountability. Educators should be recertified, i.e. retested, every decade, just as in my field, doctors are recertified every 10 years. Before the start of the school term every year, teachers should also be required to spend three weeks attending refresher courses and lectures so they can keep up to date on the latest theories in education. They should be compensated for this adult education at the same rate as their teaching salaries.

I personally know the importance of ensuring that teachers are up to par. One of my patients, a native English speaker, was a school teacher whose vocabulary was so poor she couldn't make simple conversation or understand the ramifications of her disease. The grammar and spelling on the first-visit medical history form she filled out was atrocious. One of my colleagues told me that he had the misfortune of having her as one of his high school teachers.

No. 3: Administrators should make an effort to match the subjects teachers teach with the subjects they majored in in college. This is next to impossible with math and computer and physical science majors because private industry lures them away with much more lucrative paychecks. Increased salaries for these teachers will alleviate the problem somewhat but not entirely because school budgets will never be sumptuous enough to equal corporate compensation.

No. 4: Both underperforming teachers and schools should be held accountable for their failure. They may need remedial training or in the worst case scenario—a salary cut or dismissal. Schools that consistently under perform should face the same harsh consequences and shuttered for as many years as it takes to regroup and improve. The No Child Left Behind Act provides similar sanctions for underachievers at the teaching and administrative levels.

At present, only a small percentage of parents feel the need for accountability on a national level. An *Education Week* poll in 2007 reported that a discouraging 11 percent "strongly disagree" that "to raise student achievement, low-performing schools need to be given more regulatory autonomy." That, as school performance tests already demonstrate, is a prescription for disaster. Yes, allow local school boards to continue monitoring their students and faculty, but they must also be answerable to nationwide standards, even though school administrators fear that poor results on national testing will lead to financial sanctions and teacher dismissals as prescribed by the No Child Left Behind Act of 2001.

I don't want to infringe on local schools' "autonomy;" I just want them to share it with national regulators. Local testing alone is not sufficient because many school boards "dummy down" their tests, i.e., make them easier to pass, because they are embarrassed and feel the need to cover up their students' deficiencies and show local regulators that their charges are performing well. Educators have additional motivation to demonstrate their schools' effectiveness by jerry-rigging tests because of the threat of losing Federal funding if they fail to meet standards set at the national level. To close the education gap between students in states with below average academic performance (mainly in the South) and those in states where the academic performance is higher, we must have national testing standards for all states.

No. 5: The problems of crowded classrooms and crumbling physical plants need to be addressed. The nation's schools are literally falling apart with classrooms overflowing with too many students to provide adequate instruction. In particular, libraries with limited book collections, outdated science labs and computer facilities desperately need to be upgraded. Classes need to be limited to 20 to 30 students tops. Some activists demand even less than 20 per classroom.

While demanding that the No Child Left Behind Act be scrapped, Hillary Clinton in her speech before the New York State teachers' union did agree that "proven remedies," like smaller class sizes, should be better funded than at present.

No. 6: Standardized grades for students. Just as crucial as standardized testing of students and teachers is standardized grading. By employing the same curriculum and testing nationwide, an A student in Georgia will enjoy the same academic standing as an A student in New York City, which currently is far from the case. The same will be true of failing students in Georgia and California, making it easier to identify those in peril of dropping out and provide remedial education before they ruin their lives by doing so.

Standardized grading will also make college entry more equitable and diminish what many consider is the culturally-biased and undue influence of college admission tests like the SATs and ACTs. When a student anywhere in the U.S. boasts that he's an A student, his claim will have a national reference point and a certified level of academic excellence.

No. 7: Parents should be more involved with their children's education, promote discipline at home and school, and encourage them to succeed academically. In her New York speech, Clinton also described parental involvement as one of the "proven remedies" for the low level of student achievement.

No. 8: Extra money for improving physical conditions of school and increasing teachers' salaries, especially the pay of those who teach in so-called "troubled schools" (read inner city). A poll conducted by *Educa-*

tion Week in 2006 reported that a majority of Americans, 53 percent, "strongly agree" that such teachers deserve extra remuneration for all the extra work they do inspiring underachieving students to excel. Hillary Clinton agreed with my solution and the majority of Americans when she told members of the teachers' union that they deserve greater professional respect and higher pay, especially if they were willing to work in—get ready for another liberal euphemism for the inner city—"the hardest-to-staff schools."

No More Affirmative Action

Affirmative action, the practice in which minorities with lower college entrance test scores and lower grade point averages than their Caucasian peers were shown favoritism in the admissions process at the expense of their more qualified non-minority contemporaries, has outlived its purpose.

The program began a generation ago as a way to compensate minorities for more than a century of de facto and de jure discrimination which kept them out of most white schools. Affirmation action was meant to give African Americans and other minorities a leg up the socio-economic ladder, the first leg of which is solid academic credentials.

Quotas were established that granted a set percentage of minorities admission to institutions of higher education even if their grades and test scores were inferior to white competitors'. Whether or not it was justifiable, affirmative action did work. The first executive order mandating affirmative action was signed by President John F. Kennedy in 1961, and since then the number of African Americans attending colleges and universities has doubled.

The philosophy behind affirmative action maintained that minorities were unable to compete with whites in colleges and universities due to poverty, the lack of teacher and parental encouragement, and inferior education at public schools in inner cities. To achieve the same academic and socio-economic parity, bussing was introduced at about the same time as affirmative action.

Allan Bakke, an unsuccessful white applicant to the University of California at Davis' medical school, sued after being rejected twice, claiming he had been discriminated against because he was white and that black students with inferior academic records had been admitted in his place.

In 1978, the Bakke case reached the Supreme Court, which in its traditional obfuscating way handed down a decision as equivocal and murky as its ruling on pornography, in which one Justice defined by saying, "I'll know it when I see it."

The Supreme Court ordered the University of California to admit Bakke, but it left the ruling open to future interpretation and legal challenges by declaring affirmative action "permissible but not mandatory."

When the California ballot initiative Proposition 209 in 1996 outlawed affirmative action at its prestigious University of California system, famous for its excellent academic reputation and bargain tuition compared to private colleges, the University's Board of Regents did an end run around the law and in 2001 declared that the top four percent of all graduating high school students in California were eligible for admission to the system's schools.

This allowed minority students at inferior high schools with poor SAT scores but sterling grade point averages to be admitted to the U. of C. system—and it worked. Before the Board of Regents' ruling, the absence of affirmative action dropped minority representation from 10 percent to less than one percent when admission was color-blind and only college admission test scores and G.P.A.'s were taken into account. By 2001, minority representation had jumped 17 percent and was almost at pre-Prop 209 levels.

In recent years, as in the case of bussing, affirmative action laws in many states have gradually been phased out, and I support this trend. Affirmative action is simply a recipe for reverse-discrimination and is intrinsically unfair. Americans believe in the concept of justice for all, so admission to universities should be fair and just. Admission protocols should be color-blind and not favor ethnic or religious minorities.

During their heyday, both bussing and affirmative action were justified in giving underprivileged minority groups who wanted to learn and overcome poverty and illiteracy a chance to climb the socio-economic ladder. Many minorities have taken advantage of this favoritism brilliantly. Supreme Court Justice Clarence Thomas and both of our most recent Secretaries of State, Colin L. Powell and Dr. Condoleezza Rice, were beneficiaries of affirmative action not only at the educational level but in the workplace as well.

(Liberal feminist detractors who condemned Justice Thomas for his alleged sexual harassment of aide Anita Hill reluctantly conceded that Thomas, who falls asleep during afternoon sessions of the Supreme Court and rarely asks questions during testimony, was an embarrassing example of the failure of affirmative action because Thomas, with his less than sterling judicial résumé, was not qualified to hold the highest position in the U.S. Justice system. His mediocre record on the Court and slacker behavior reinforces that assessment.)

Many other minority success stories—CEOs, doctors, attorneys, elected officials—are due to affirmative action, but these beneficiaries now reject affirmative action for their own children because it questions a minority's legitimate achievements and dismisses them as the unearned result of affirmative action. These successful professionals also don't feel the need for affirmative action because they can afford to send their children to the best private schools or pay their transportation to superior suburban public schools.

But minorities who after almost half a century of affirmative action in one form or another still haven't grasped the brass ring of socio-economic success offered by quota systems favoring minorities need a more effective alternative to affirmative action. Increased parental involvement is the key to ending minorities' failure. Families must provide an environment that encourages academic excellence and downplays athletic prowess—all enforced by strict discipline in the home, which will carry over into good behavior at school. Drug-and gun-free homes will lead to drug-and gun-free schools.

Discipline and encouragement will allow minority students to catch the train of educational advancement which will lead to gratifying careers without relying on artificial and unfair quota systems, especially with this work's recommended standardization of school curricula and testing on a nationwide basis so that schools in the Deep South will be as academically qualified as their counterparts in the more affluent regions of the nation.

Asian Americans are good examples of how parental involvement can make affirmative action unnecessary. Asian children are entering Ivy League colleges and other top academic institutions in numbers greater than their representation in the general population without relying on quota systems. The reason is that their families have programmed them to strive for scholastic excellence and even perfectionism. They set high standards for their children to reach the top ... and they do.

Many Asian-American families make financial sacrifices to provide their children with excellent college-prep educations. They order their offspring not to engage in disruptive behavior at school and not join the crowd of student losers known as "slackers" and "druggies." (A University of Michigan study in 2000 said that 54 percent of high school seniors use drugs.) These parents encourage their children to "stay the course" and not drop out of school for a low-paying, dead-end job.

Family participation has not only helped Asian—American students. Other minority group children also excel in school, and this is due to family guidance and financial sacrifice. This is particularly true of the children of recent immigrants. Their children are inspired by their parents' determination to achieve despite such huge handicaps as illegal immigrant status, lack of formal education and poor or non-existent job skills.

School Vouchers, the Left Wing's *Bête Noire*

If you want to see liberals foam at the mouth, bring up the subject of school vouchers, which would give cash grants to parents who want to opt out of the deteriorating public school system and send their children to private schools instead. Opponents of vouchers claim that the program would drain money away from already under funded public schools, and they also make the First Amendment argument that paying for religious school tuition does not maintain the separation of church and state.

Advocates of vouchers, mainly conservative Protestants and most Catholics, love the idea of subsidizing private schools because many of them already send their children to faith-based or parochial schools. Of course, non-denominational private schools would also be eligible for vouchers, thus taking the wind out of the First Amendment-based objections.

School vouchers will not drain money from Federal coffers if they are non-discriminatory and offered to all socio-economic classes, the rich, the middle class and the poor, just as Medicare is provided for everyone at age 65 regardless of his or her financial status. Rich and poor alike support the public school system by paying Federal and local taxes. But in this rare instance, it's the rich, not the poor, who are being ripped off by unfair taxes. The rich pay more in taxes than the middle class and the poor to fund public schools, but they receive no benefit from this tax burden because so many of them send their children to private schools, losing all the tax money they contribute to public education.

I sent my own children to private schools even though I paid a substantial portion of my income in taxes for the upkeep of public schools. I recommend cash subsidies of $5,000 for parents with children who are privately educated, which is still only a fraction of the average tuition of $30,000 per year that private, non-denominational schools charge their affluent patrons. If the middle class and even the poor care to enroll their children in private schools, they can opt for less prestigious (and much cheaper) schools where a $5,000 subsidy will go a much longer way.

The upper middle class, if they are really interested in seeing their children get ahead, may use the $5,000 vouchers as a partial reimbursement that will allow them to enroll their kids in pricier and more prestigious non-denominational schools that boast greater academic excellence than faith-based institutions. The most prestigious of these college-prep schools virtually guarantee all but its dimmest bulbs entré to the Ivy Leagues. John F. Kennedy attended the non-denominational Choate Academy, where he was an average student ranked 62 out of a class of 112. Despite his academic mediocrity, he went on to Harvard. Our current President, after two years in public high school in Texas, transferred to the elite Andover Academy, his father's alma mater, which undoubtedly helped the younger Bush, a C-student with unimpressive SAT scores (566 verbal, 640 math), gain admission to Yale, also his father's alma mater, where he continued to earn C's, and then on to Harvard's graduate business school. *Slate*, the on-line magazine, referred to Bush's acceptance into his father's alma maters as the "Ivy Leagues' Affirmative-Action program for alumni brats."

Private religious schools, especially parochial ones, already in effect subsidize parents by charging them less than the actual cost of educating their children—with the difference made up by the collection plate passed around during Sunday Mass—although these days more and more of the collection plate seems to go toward legal expenses and punitive damages paid to the victims of pedophile priests.

As for the First Amendment argument against vouchers, if public schools, especially those that serve the underprivileged, do suffer a loss of funding to private schools, I recommend an unobjectionable increase in Federal Income taxes of no more than one percent.

CHAPTER SEVEN
Saving Us From Criminals

Just as it is the right of every American citizen to have access to affordable health care and a quality education for his or her children, it is also the right of everyone in the U.S. to go anywhere without fear of any internal (street or household crime) or external (domestic terrorism) threat. It is the duty of elected government officials, the police and the judiciary to protect their citizens from crime and punish every convicted criminal.

Unfortunately, the government is not fulfilling its duty to protect its citizens, and the U.S. is not a safe place, especially when compared to Europe, Canada, Australia and such industrialized Asian nations as Japan, South Korea, Singapore (which imprisons drug dealers and their customers for life) and China (which stands embezzlers and purse-snatchers up against a firing squad in a stadium filled with spectators).

Strict laws and the certainty of swift punishment deter crime. I have visited Singapore twice, and on one occasion, the captain of my plane did a curious thing. Over the public address system, like a society hostess offering her guests a crucial etiquette tip, the captain before landing reminded all passengers of the harsh anti-narcotics laws of the island nation and urged them to leave any illicit drugs behind on the plane before disembarking because if caught, they faced life behind bars.

In 2006, a young Australian woman didn't heed the pilot's advice and was arrested in Singapore for bringing a tiny amount of marijuana into the country and received the maximum penalty of life imprisonment. The rest of the world condemned Singapore for imposing such a major penalty on such a minor crime, but the authorities ignored pleas to free her.

Street crime in Saudi Arabia is virtually non-existent, and it's not a coincidence that is among the nations with the harshest penalties for even minor offenses. Ironically, Saudis are adherents of their Jewish nemeses' Mosaic law—an eye for an eye, a tooth for a tooth, a life for a life. If you take a life, you lose yours. Muggers are "encouraged" not to assault victims with the realization that if caught, they will lose the hand that perpetrated the crime. In effect, convicted purse-snatchers receive a life sentence of one-handedness.

Sometimes, however, it is hard to compute equivalent punishment for the crime committed. Rapists can't be raped, so in Saudi Arabia they are stoned to death instead. Punishment is not only severe but swift and inescapable. Beating even Saddam Hussein's record of fast "justice," Saudi Arabia executes convicted criminals within 30 days of their conviction. While I don't agree with the harshness of Saudi law which is based on the Koran and not on a constitution, Saudi Arabia remains safer than any big city in the so-called civilized world.

The only major difference between the U.S. and other industrialized nations—other than our inferior healthcare system—is that they ban guns and none of their constitutions contains the equivalent of our toxic Second Amendment that purportedly allows private gun ownership.

Drastic acts of violence are frequent and are overwhelming a traumatized nation, forced to watch endless replays on TV of footage of the mass murders for weeks after they occur. I began composing this chapter a few days after the Virginia Tech massacre, in which a paranoid schizophrenic student gunned down 32 peers and faculty before turning the gun on himself—the highest casualty figure in the history of U.S. mass murders.

While Virginia Tech was the most sanguine example of large-scale carnage, it is not rare and mass murderers have almost as long a history as the history of this country itself. Gunmen have gone on rampages at Columbine High, the West Nickel Mines Amish School in Pennsylvania, and the Universities of Texas and Virginia. Crazed murderers do not confine themselves to institutions of higher learning. So many disgruntled U.S. Post Office employees have annihilated co-workers that the phrase "going postal," i.e., going crazy and murdering your colleagues, has entered the national vocabulary, although in fairness it should be noted that studies show postal workers do not commit mass murder at a higher rate than any other occupations. We're not even safe at that shrine to inexpensive American consumerism, Wal-Mart, which has seen its share of blood-letting in the store aisles.

Fatalities, of course, aren't restricted to high body counts. It seems that almost every day the media reports on yet another one or two victims of deadly gunplay. European and Canadian cities have a microscopic homicide rate compared to the U.S.—if you don't count recent terrorist attacks there, which have especially traumatized the citizens of those previously peaceful cities because they simply aren't used to violent crime. It's as freak an occurrence as though a mob of *jihadis* suddenly descended on Disney World or suicide bombers invested Dollywood.

While President Bush largely won reelection in 2004 because Americans believed he would best protect them from another domestic terror attack like 9/11, such attacks are the rare exception. The norm is *home-grown* violence, not clueless shoe bombers who can't figure out how to light a match to blow up an airliner.

After a horrific event like Virginia Tech, crime prevention briefly boils over on the front burner as the media keeps busy rebroadcasting videotape of the bloody scenes and asking experts if gun ownership, society, lenient criminal sentencing laws and even permissive parenting are to blame for the mayhem.

Or is violence simply the American way of life and death—an atavism that has survived from our frontier days when vigilante justice stepped into the vacuum created by the lack of law enforcement officials and often represented legitimate survival tactics not random viciousness?

Following a national trauma like Virginia Tech or Columbine, gun control becomes a hot issue—for a while—but Americans have a notorious short attention span, and after a brief period of mourning and Monday-morning quarterbacking, people are distracted by Paris Hilton's latest DUI or Alec Baldwin's atrocious telephone manners.

Courtesy of the NRA and its paid political supporters, Republicans in our state and national legislatures, gun ownership is promoted as an inalienable right guaranteed by the Second Amendment to the U.S. Constitution, which is maddeningly ambiguous as to whether the amendment allows private citizens or only local militia (like the police) to bear arms.

The NRA's Republican lackeys don't care that guns kill adults, but they obsess about abortion killing fetuses. Liberal Democratic legislators so far have kept abortion rights legal, but only barely, and they remain silent on the issue of gun control, fearful that the mighty war chest of the NRA will finance their opponents' campaigns in the next race and lead to defeat, which has happened so often that Democrats seem downright phobic about uttering the "g" word.

Craven gun control advocates in Congress don't speak up because they want to remain in office indefinitely, considering their jobs a life-time career opportunity, not a limited time to spend serving one's country—then stepping aside to let fresh blood and fresh ideas see if they can solve America's intractable problems. That's why Chapter One was so adamant about term limits for both the executive and legislative branches of the Federal government. An obsession by elected officials to hold on to their jobs at any cost also often leads to corruption as desperate office-holders succumb to the financial blandishments (read bribes) of lobbyists and the special interests who employ them.

For inexplicable reasons, most churches also fail to criticize the NRA even though priests and ministers don't face reelection to their ministries every two to six years, and the NRA isn't a big contributor to church collection plates. Church leaders—priests and ministers—must come out of holy hibernation and remind their flock that killing is a sin. They need to remind them of that little ordinance in the Old Testament called the Sixth Commandment. And that the easiest and most effective way to violate that commandment is by using a gun.

Instead, some pastors—usually on the extreme fringes of the Christian right—actively encourage their congregants to violate the Sixth Commandment when they urge them to assassinate foreign dictators with a leftist or atheistic bent. The Reverend Pat Robertson is both paranoid and grandiose—or is it just early Alzheimer's?—when he makes lunatic suggestions like taking out Venezuela strongman Hugo Chavez. In a 2005 broadcast of his program, *The 700 Club*, the televangelist said, "… if he thinks we're trying to assassinate him, I think that we really ought to go ahead and do it. It's a whole lot cheaper than starting a war. We have the ability to take him out, and I think the time has come that we exercise that ability. We don't need another $200 billion war to get rid of one … strong-arm dictator. It's a whole lot easier to have some of the covert operatives do the job and then get it over with."

If the President of Venezuela is such a menace, let his own people take care of the problem through the ballot box or the barrel of a gun—just as long as that gun is not wielded by some crazed American follower of some crazed American churchman.

Gun manufacturers only care about profits at any cost—even at the cost of innocent lives, offering up the indefensible bromide/cliché that "guns don't kill people, *people* kill people." What they conveniently neglect to add is that only people *with guns* kill people. (OK, knives, ropes, poison, and even fists also contribute to the death toll, but there are no multi-billion-dollar lobbies promoting their manufacture.)

Many culprits have been blamed for bleeding America. Is it due to our violent culture turbocharged by dramatic presentations of homicides on TV and in films? Is strong lobbying by the NRA a major contributor to violent crime? Is it due to weak or nonexistent gun-control laws? Are there just too many evil or mentally impaired people among the population? Does most churches' shameful silence on gun control and media violence allow people of faith to ignore the urgency of the issue? Are the media pimping for Nielsen ratings and CD sales by using violence as a marketing tool? Or does a weak judicial system with no guaranteed and swift punishment fail to deter criminal behavior? Unfortunately, all of the above miscreants share the blame for our toxic culture.

Maybe the NRA is right and guns are not the cause of our Wild West lawlessness. The NRA maintains that gun-control laws are futile because there are already millions of guns on the street in this country, so even with strict gun control or an outright ban on these weapons, criminals will still have access to the guns already in circulation.

Gun-control advocates may be focusing on the wrong guilty party. Evil people do need guns to kill innocent citizens, but guns need bullets. Without them, they are as lethal as water pistols or bean shooters. Instead of banning guns, which isn't going to happen as long as the NRA keeps buying Congressmen, we need to ban bullets. Make it illegal to manufacture them. If it remains impossible to ban guns, then ban gun factories. Shutter all of them except government facilities that make weapons for law enforcement officers and keep those facilities under strict supervision so that there is no "leakage"—i.e., no corrupt cops selling government-manufactured guns to criminals on the black market.

It may take the passing of an entire generation to break people of the habit of owning handguns and buying bullets, but eventually, the market and the mentality that supports it will evaporate in the next 10 to 20 years. In time, we will reverse the arc of violence instead of escalating it.

How many more massacres like Virginia Tech, Columbine and similar bloodbaths will it take before we wake up and smell the gunpowder, change our attitude toward guns, keep our families safe by limiting the number of guns in circulation by limiting their manufacture and by shutting down factories that make bullets?

The NRA and other gun advocates argue that strict laws in one state are ineffective because criminals will just cross the border and make their purchases in states with laxer gun control enforcement, but fatality statistics undercut this argument. New York state and others have strict gun control legislation, and their murder rate from firearms is much lower than in nearby states like Virginia, which is a gun fancier's paradise.

Pop culture is No. 1 on my hit list of what turbocharges violence in our society. As soon as an infant is able to open his eyes, he sees violence splattered all over the airwaves and movie theaters. As the child matures and develops digital dexterity, ultra violent and unregulated videogames reinforce the bloody images on TV and in film.

Rap music that encourages killing police, "hos" and even annoying girlfriends metastasizes throughout our culture via CDs, DVDS, radio and TV. Rap popularizes the degradation of women in obscene detail and desensitizes its fans, which consumer surveys show the majority of whom are white, middle-class suburban teenage boys! Ebonics is the language of disaffected white youths. Rap's frequent *jihads* urging listeners to kill da police and honkeys stimulate similar desensitization.

What the First Amendment Is Not

The Federal government through legislation and executive decrees should protect our children from the malign influence of violence proffered by film, TV, radio and the recording industry. The First Amendment guarantees freedom of speech to express political views and religious beliefs. The amendment does not allow the "freedom" to incite rape, kill police and make substance abuse and excessive alcohol consumption glamorous just as a famous Supreme Court ruling said that shouting "FIRE!" in a crowded theater wasn't covered by the amendment either.

That's not freedom; it's called conspiracy to commit crime, a punishable offense, just as child predators are busted for trying to make assignations with minors even though, according to an *Los Angeles Times* report, 70 percent of "minors" on the other end of the Internet conversation are undercover vice cops. No child has been harmed by the predator in those undercover sting operations, just as rap lyrics or violent films in and of themselves do not literally kill people. But their intention to harm and kill should be punishable by law. The First Amendment does not give adults carte blanche to harm children by speech or deed.

Our children grow and fester in an environment polluted with moral and cultural garbage. Parents are too disengaged to monitor what their children are watching, playing or listening to. They shell out big bucks so their kids can own the latest in videogame mayhem without bothering to check what the computer games depict. In 1992, when Tipper Gore, Al's wife, simply suggested rating, not censoring, rap albums based on their lyrics so parents wouldn't have to spare the time listening to the dissonant music, she was practically accused by First Amendment zealots of promoting Nazi-style book burnings.

The Internet is also doing its part to corrupt our youth—not to mention desperate child predators. In the past 15 to 20 years, cyberspace has created a parallel universe that exposes children to pornography, criminal activity, gun and drug use and even bomb-making! Instead of doing homework, adolescents spend hours after school obliterating bad guys on their computer monitors.

At school, they are exposed to the criminal mentality of fellow students who introduce them to guns, knives and drugs—and where to buy them. These human crime waves often become role models—"kewl," as teens spell it—and innocent children begin to emulate their malign peers'

pathologies. Again, thanks to the instant gratification of the Internet, these toxic ideas spread from child to child literally at the speed of light.

Sometimes students don't need to get their guns from classmates. Often without their parents' knowledge, they expropriate the family firearms—yet another reason gun control advocates want to ban private ownership because legally owned weapons can still end up in the wrong hands, such as children's. Parents must monitor their children after school not only to make sure they finish their homework and don't spend too much time frying their brains with ultra violent videogames, but also to keep them out of the family gun rack, which should be kept locked at all time.

Parents need to be aware if their children are hiding drugs in the home or purloining firearms from the family armory. To make them more accountable for their children's behavior, parents should be prosecuted and pay a big penalty—financial or penal, depending on the severity of their offsprings' misdeeds—for failing to secure weapons in the home.

Before the women's movement of the 1960s, dad went to work and mom stayed home and prevented the kids away from brandishing pistols at school, among other domestic chores. Today, both parents tend to work, and latch-key children return home while their parents are still at the office. This leaves them free to be bombarded by violent rap lyrics and images on TV and Play Stations. They mature in an environment of virtual violence.

Children are notorious copycats and famously susceptible to peer-group pressure. When those peers are gun, drug and alcohol aficionados, who also happen to be members of the "in" group at school, they become irresistible role models, and innocent students are sucked into their universe of destructive behavior. Students also don't respect one another, especially when it comes to the opposite sex. My friends tell me that 30 years ago boys and girls treated one another with courtesy. Now, it's "kewl" to insult and sexually harass girls.

The Second Amendment—Carte Blanche for Gun Ownership?

"A well regulated militia, being necessary to the security of a free state, the right of the people to keep and bear arms, shall not be infringed."

Who could have predicted that a single simple sentence in a 220-year-old document would result in the gun-related deaths of 30,708 Americans every year, according to a 1998 report by the National Academy of Sciences' Institute of Medicine?

The United States leads the industrialized world in firearms violence of all types—homicides, suicides, and unintentional deaths, the National Center for Health Statistics in Maryland reported in 1998.

As discussed in a previous chapter, gun enthusiasts take advantage of the Second Amendment quoted above to justify gun ownership by private citizens, even though our Founding Fathers tacked the amendment on to the U.S. Constitution in 1787 to guarantee the rights of "militias," i.e., volunteer citizen soldiers, to bear arms specifically to protect the out-gunned colonists/revolutionaries against the well-armed invading British army.

The framers of the Constitution intended the amendment to put weapons in the hands of revolutionaries not late-night liquor store bandits. During the American Revolution and the War of 1812, the first and last time the continental U.S. was violated by foreigners until 9/11, the regular army and citizen militias protected non-combatants.

Today, every American civilian is a non-combatant except for criminals, and the duty of keeping law-abiding Americans safe from these "combatants" rests with law enforcement officers, not gun-toting vigilantes who statistically use their weapons more often against family and friends instead of burglars and muggers.

According to the Violence Policy Center, a Washington, D.C.-based gun-control advocacy group, only 1.3 percent of handgun homicides in 1997 were committed by strangers. Most victims know their killers, who are often relatives. And Americans not only need protection from lethal loved ones, but also from themselves. In a 1988 article, the *American Journal of Public Health* noted that the weapon of choice of suicide victims— 70 percent of them—was a handgun.

In his 1994 book, *Stopping Power*, criminologist J. Neil Schulman claimed that 70 million Americans own guns, while a report from the National Opinion Research Center (NORC) at the University of Chicago in 2000 stated that only 25 percent of Americans were handgun owners and 37 percent favor a "law that would ban possession of handguns except for the police and other authorized persons." (Not surprisingly, the same study said that in crime-stricken New York City, almost 70 percent of residents favor a total ban.)

Further research, however, needs to be done: 1) Big city police departments should determine how many criminals were killed by legal gun owners in self-defense. 2) How many innocent victims have been killed by criminals with handguns and 3) How many people were killed by family members in the same household? These studies will once and for all settle the argument whether or not guns protect the innocent from criminals and whether or not the presence of guns in the home increases the likelihood of one family member offing another.

If our forefathers had been able to foresee that the Second Amendment would be used as a justification to kill their fellow Americans, they would have rewritten it more precisely so that it allowed only militias the right to bear arms. If they had known about Columbine and Virginia Tech, *et al.*, they might have excluded it from the Bill of Rights altogether.

Firearms are ubiquitous and deeply embedded in American culture and commerce. You can pick them up at gun shops, department stores, gun shows, flea markets and even K-Mart and Wal-Mart, along with a gallon of milk and a toaster oven.

The NRA among other gun ownership advocates claims that background criminal checks will keep guns out of the hands of criminals. Not true. This is self-evident: a criminal has no record before he commits his first crime. The perpetrators of both the Columbine and Virginia Tech bloodbaths had no criminal background before they went hunting classmates.

Even someone with a criminal record can circumvent the background check by purchasing his weapons at gun shows or flea markets, which are not required by law to conduct such checks. These venues also have no waiting period; you can buy your gun on the spot, a boon for those who kill on impulse. If a prospective gun owner lives in a state with relatively strict gun control laws, he can simply drive across the border to a state with more lenient enforcement. The argument that there are laws on the books providing some control is moot after the killing has already taken place.

What especially enrages me is that after a major incident like Virginia Tech or Columbine, pro-gun advocates (e.g., Newt Gingrich) claim that if everyone had been armed at the university or high school or anywhere else for that matter, prospective shooters would be prevented from committing their crimes because they would be shot by other gun-toting students before they got the chance to cock their pistols.

Even more ludicrous is the suggestion, originally made as a joke by Archie Bunker on the 1970s sit-com *All in the Family*, that all passengers on airplanes should be packing a sidearm to foil terrorist hijackings. Imagine 250 amateurs, untrained, frazzled by fear and panic, firing away in the close quarters of an airline cabin. They would cause more fatalities than the hijackers. If this insane reasoning is taken to its logical extreme, passengers boarding a plane would be handed guns and knives instead of having them confiscated.

If I knew of a college or high school where all the students were packing, I wouldn't let my children go there. What if a fight erupts in a classroom or hallway—or in a movie theater, bar or shopping mall? With firearms, what would have turned into a fistfight could degenerate into the biggest massacre in the history of the U.S. with participants shooting indiscriminately at each other the way bar brawlers take swings at other patrons without knowing whose side they're on.

What kind of Damoclean sword would hang above the heads of school teachers who realize every one of their students is a possible assassin if they don't like the grade they got on a test. In that situation, sending the gunman to the principal's office is not an option.

Proponents of semi-automatic assault rifles like AK-47s are the looniest. Of what possible use would such a bulky firearm be in the case of a close-quarter encounter with a mugger who's in your face? Or a rapist pressed tight up against his victim? The NRA claims machineguns are for shooting wild animals, not humans, even though police officer associations consistently call for their ban because criminals are often better armed than lawmen. Hunters may keep their rifles—when they're hunting. The rest of the time, their weapons should be locked up in a well-guarded storehouse like the Beverly Hills Gun Club.

Some gun-control advocates are more zealous than I. California's Democratic Senator Diane Feinstein and New York's Charles Schumer and Hillary Clinton passed the Federal Assault Weapons Ban of 1994 in response to a mass shooting in 1993 at a law firm in Feinstein's hometown of San Francisco.

When the law was due to expire 10 years later, 74 percent of Americans—including a surprising 50 percent of gun owners—wanted Congress and the President to renew it, according to a 2003 survey by the Consumer Federation of America, but it was allowed to lapse by a Republican-controlled Congress in September 2004.

In fact, whenever any member of Congress, almost always a Democrat, proposes a similar ban on assault weapons or even just limiting their availability, the NRA and their partners in crime enabling trot out the Second Amendment while reaching deep into their pockets to buy other Congressmen who will vote against gun-control legislation. This relatively small interest group has successfully blocked most gun control legislation despite the fact that three-fourths of Americans desire some form of it.

Although the police tend to lean right on every other political issue, they and the head of the FBI in most big cities favor strict gun control for the simple reason that they don't want to fight an enemy often better armed than they are.

The fate of handgun ownership and other lethal weapons should be left in the hands of the American people. That is why in Chapter One a national referendum to decide this matter and others once and for all was so strongly urged. The results of such a referendum are a no-brainer if it is indeed true that as many as 75 percent of voters want to ban or limit fire-arm possession.

If citizens have a change of heart or the polls are inaccurate and they vote against a ban, the same referendum can determine which groups—students or psychos, fathers or serial rapists—can and cannot possess weapons that cause major destruction—not to mention killing Bambi's mother.

Prior to a national referendum, there should be an open debate and dis-cussion free from the influence of special interest groups, plus educational seminars on crime, guns and related topics. Then let the American people decide in the referendum whether they prefer the status quo or the liquida-tion of firearms.

It's not too outrageous an analogy to maintain that the disproportionate amount of influence wielded by a tiny percentage of Americans—lobbyists and their special interest financiers—resemble Afghanistan's Taliban sociopaths where a small number of Talibs once dominated an entire country, enforcing a 1,400-year-old misogynist culture and customs in which women were treated like second-class citizens, prohibiting the edu-cation of girls, disenfranchising women in general and forcing them to wear in an Equatorial climate suffocating burkas whose tiny peepholes cause purblindness.

The assertion that evil people, not evil guns, kill people is countered by the argument that if there were no evil guns, evil people wouldn't possess them. The lack of effective gun control differentiates America from all other industrialized nations, a difference that has often been explained by the claim that the U.S. still possesses a frontier mentality where horse thieves were hanged and differences of opinion were settled by shootouts in the center of Downtown Dodge.

In the rest of the industrialized world, only the police are armed. In fact, until 35 years ago, British Bobbies were only allowed to carry night-sticks. Only the special forces comparable to America's SWAT teams packed pistols. Over the past three decades, policemen in the U.K. have been allowed to carry guns because terrorists acts perpetuated by immi-grants—mostly from Commonwealth countries whose citizens are allowed unrestricted entry to the U.K.—started to become common.

Britain's experience and reaction to mass murder proves that gun con-trol laws work. In 1996, after 16 students and a teacher were killed in Dunblane, Scotland by a lone gunman—a defrocked Boy Scout leader, Tony Blair's government abolished the possession of handguns by all citi-zens. There have been no mass murders in Scotland since.

Our Flawed Judicial System

For every "hanging judge" who sentences 7–11 shoplifters to 20 years in prison for stealing a $1.25 candy bar, there are bleeding heart jurists who coddle criminals. The latter do not punish serious crimes severely enough and are deaf to the outcry of gun victims who often see their assailant get off on a technicality or for lack of evidence.

It's a national disgrace that more jails and prisons aren't being con-structed, and the result is that vicious criminals are released early or with no time spent behind bars at all because of overcrowded and understaffed penal institutions. It's a safe bet that the American people would approve a one-percent increase in Federal income taxes to build more prisons and hire more guards.

There are too many laws to protect the rights of defendants and not enough to protect the rights of their victims. Civil liberty advocates and the liberal media care more about criminals than crime victims and worry more about the perpetrators' rights being violated. After conviction, criminals should have no rights, and our concerns and financial restitution should focus on the victims and their families.

Justice is supposed to be blind, but punishment rarely is. Unequal justice causes a dramatic disparity in retribution. If two individuals commit the same crime, their sentences will depend on the whether the judge is right-or left-leaning, the quality of the defense lawyers and the often illogical legal reasoning of jurors who are amateurs and who should not be deciding technical points of law that might baffle a law professor.

In Sweden, jurors are professionals with years of training in jurisprudence, not Joe Blow randomly selected from an unwilling pool of jurors showing up only under duress. Justice is not blind when it comes to money or race. Rich defendants, most notoriously white collar criminals, suffer much less severe penalties than indigents represented for free by mediocre public defenders. Some clichés are indeed true: you get (or lose) what you pay for.

Until the recent Federal crackdown on white collar crime, accused business executives surrendering to authorities were allowed to sneak in the back door of the courthouse for finger-printing, mug shots, etc. Now they are forced to do the same "perp walk" that violent criminals are subjected to—handcuffed and frog-marched through the front door, their disgrace and humiliation recorded by TV cameras and broadcast to the entire nation.

To deter potential white collar criminals, those convicted of juggling their companies' profit/loss reports to stockholders or bribing Congressmen should know that they will receive a mandatory minimum 10-year prison sentence and that there is no parole in the Federal prison system. Ten years means ten years, not five years because he was such a great … fill in the blank: father, son, colleague, philanthropist, legislator.

The possessions of these non-violent criminals should all be confiscated along with their bank accounts and stock portfolios, which often contain hundreds of millions of dollars ripped off from elderly pensioners whose retirement nest egg has evaporated along with the value of the stock they own in bankrupt companies like Enron. If felony-minded executives realize that they will lose everything, not just their personal freedom but all the money that prompted them to commit their crimes in the first place, they may think twice before cheating unsophisticated Native Americans out of their casino profits or taking Congressmen on junkets to exotic foreign golf courses.

A much more dangerous kind of criminal presents an even more intractable problem: What to do with the percentage of child molesters known as "predators," recidivists who after release from prison go on to molest and/or murder again and again. More than one study has shown that such recidivists receive no benefit from counseling, Sex Addicts Anonymous meetings or other treatment programs.

For this species of societal monster, we need a new "*two* strikes and you're out" law. For the first offense, the should receive a lengthy prison sentence if for no other reason—since prison doesn't serve as a deterrent to these repeat offenders—than to keep them away from future child victims as long as a liberal court system will allow. After a second offense and conviction, they return to prison—for keeps.

But everyone deserves a chance at redemption, even child rapists who murder their victims to eliminate the only witness to their crime, and early release should be offered to those who after serving a suitably long punitive sentence if they agree to be castrated. As heartless as this sounds, I recommend physical rather than chemical castration. The latter procedure uses drugs like estrogen (female hormones) that have proven to be carcinogenic, but even more important, once the chemically castrated sex offender is released, he may stop injecting the female hormones, which have creepy side effects like gynecomastia (male breast development). Physical castration is, like two strikes and you're out, for keeps.

Race, Juries and the Death Penalty

White jurors often refuse to convict white police officers despite videotape evidence of them beating the hell out of inner city blacks, while primarily black juries let celebrities and convicted felons like O.J. Simpson literally get away with murder that others who can't afford high-priced legal counsel are executed for.

Arguments both for and against the death penalty are seductive, and it's difficult to decide which position is more defensible. Some believe the death penalty is an effective deterrent, while others point to studies that show criminals never even think about the possibility of being put to death while they're preoccupied with putting their victims to death. Death penalty opponents enjoy citing the 18th century phenomenon in which pickpockets were publicly hanged to deter other pickpockets. During these supposedly deterring executions, spectators often had their pockets picked.

Recent scholarly analyses show that the threat of being put to death does serve as a deterrent. In 2003, a study at the University of Colorado at Denver, followed by a reexamination of the data in 2006, contended that each execution prevents five homicides, while commuting a death sentence causes five more.

Ironically, the co-author of the studies, a University of Colorado economics professor, Naci Mocan, is a strong opponent of the death penalty, but felt compelled to publish the results of his research. "There is no question about it. The conclusion is that it does have a deterrent effect. I oppose the death penalty. But my results show that the death penalty deters. What am I going to do? Hide [the results]?

Other studies confirm Professor Mocan's conclusions. According to a nationwide study conducted by Emory University in 2003, for each execution that takes place, 18 homicides are prevented. After Illinois suspended the death sentence 150 additional murders were committed, according to a 2006 study conducted at the University of Houston.

Critics claim that these studies made serious mistakes in methodology and that there are too few executions per year to prove a connection between deterrence and the homicide rate. In 2005, 60 executions were carried out. "We just don't have enough data to say anything," said Justin Wolfers, an economics professor at the University of Pennsylvania's Wharton School of Business, who in 2006 published a critique of these studies, which he categorized as "flimsy" and dismissed as being published by "second-tier journals."

The death penalty is also no bargain. A death sentence automatically mandates a series of appeals that keep murderers on death row for an average of 10 to 20 years. The thrifty argue why should we spend thousands of tax dollars keeping child rapist/murderers locked up for life, but one study estimated that it costs on average $500,000 to incarcerate a convict forever, while the endless legal appeals for all those sentenced to death are entitled to cost on average $1.5 million. Lawyers don't come cheap, even relatively low-salaried public defenders who handle the majority of death penalty appeals.

There are two ways to deal with the death penalty: abolish it or speed up the process from conviction to lethal injection. As much as it may pain one to admit it, Saddam Hussein got at least one thing right: Ironically a victim of his own system, Saddam while he was in power allowed 30 days of appeals after a conviction for a capital crime and another 30 days before punishment was carried out. Sixty days after his own conviction, he was swinging from a rope amid taunts from Shiites he had persecuted for decades. In Egypt and in much of the rest of the Middle East, punishment is almost as swift as in Iraq. Within three months of conviction, the defendant meets his Maker.

A 2004 study by Emory University confirms my contention that swift and certain punishment acts as a deterrent. According to the Emory study, one murder is prevented for every 2.75 years cut from the time the condemned spends on death row.

Opponents of capital punishment like to reference studies showing that after the 1987 introduction of DNA testing in the U.S., many prisoners sent to their deaths were innocent. In a study conducted between 1995 and 1996 and cited by the on-line *Crime* magazine, which bills itself as "an encyclopedia of crime," researchers found that 28 people indicted but not convicted of a capital offense could not have committed their alleged crimes because of DNA evidence exonerating them.

That's 28 people who might have met the business end of a syringe filled with poisons. Statistics like those shocked the former Republican governor of Illinois, George Ryan, formerly a big death penalty advocate, into indefinitely suspending the sentences of everyone on death row in Illinois as of January 2003.

Opponents also justify ending the death penalty because they claim that it falls under the U.S. Constitution's typically vague description of "cruel and unusual punishment." California Governor Arnold Schwarzenegger, the Golden State's answer to Rudy Giuliani—a closet liberal in a conservative Republican's clothing—suspended the death sentence in his state after deciding that it was indeed cruel, even though like most states, California uses the allegedly painless form of execution, lethal injection.

Proponents of the death penalty insist that lethal injection is not painful, as anyone who has ever been knocked out by an anesthesiologist just before being wheeled into the operating room knows. But their argument is faulty. The anesthesiologist doesn't use two of the drugs the executioner uses, which are supposedly extremely painful. The first drug injected, sodium pentothal, a barbiturate that belongs to the same family of drugs that did Marilyn Monroe and Judy Garland in, just puts the convicted to sleep, the same way your kindly anesthesiologist prepares you for the surgeon's scalpel.

Regular pre-op patients receive 100 to 150 milligrams. The condemned receive as much as 5,000 milligrams, which according to HowStuff-Works.com, is a lethal dosage and at the very least, proponents of the death penalty insist that after the sodium pentothal is injected, the inmate doesn't feel anything. But it's the next two injected chemicals that do the dirty work, pancuronium bromide and potassium chloride, the former a muscle relaxant that causes pulmonary arrest by paralyzing the lungs and diaphragm and the latter, potassium chloride, causes cardiac arrest.

The dosage for sodium pentothal varies dramatically from state to state, with some states using half the dose that others employ. At the lower dosage, opponents of the procedure claim, the inmate is not completely anesthetized or rendered unconscious and feels the next two drugs, which are excruciatingly painful. That argument prompted Governor Schwarzenegger to suspend the death penalty as cruel and unusual.

But based on my own experience as a nephrologist (kidney specialist) and internist, I believe that even at the lower dosage sodium pentothal completely anesthetizes the patient, and even if it doesn't, potassium chloride does not cause a painful or "cruel and unusual" death. Many of my heart and kidney patients have accidentally been killed by nurses who incorrectly prescribe potassium chloride in larger doses than necessary.

Sometimes, a patient is kept on a small dose of potassium chloride, which is safely cleared by the kidneys. But when kidney failure occurs, the organ can't flush the potassium chloride, and if the infusion of potassium chloride isn't stopped immediately, the patient's heart stops beating.

I have personally witnessed such accidental deaths, and the victim dies painlessly. Indeed, I recommend that executioners only use potassium chloride and skip the other two drugs as unneeded. The same drug and delivery system, potassium chloride via intravenous infusion, was used by "Dr. Death," Jack Kevorkian, in his physician-assisted suicides while his patient was conscious, and no pain was reported as the terminally ill individual slid into unconsciousness and finally death.

As for DNA evidence demonstrating the innocence of so many inmates on death row, I would only advocate the death penalty for those whose guilt has been proven beyond a reasonable doubt either through the impeccable testimony of eyewitnesses or better yet, a confession by the killer, or positive DNA evidence—two of the three justify the death penalty. Does anybody doubt that if the Virginia Tech student had not committed suicide a jury would have failed to convict him of the massacre?

In cases where the alleged witness' claims are suspicious because he's a convicted criminal himself who has been offered a plea bargain for his perjured testimony and who often later recants, I am of course opposed to the death penalty. Also in the absence of a confession by the accused, the ultimate punishment should not be inflicted. The case must be clear-cut and unequivocal before the death penalty is imposed.

Privacy Laws Protect the Mentally Ill But Endanger the General Population

In 1996, Congress passed the HIPAA (Health Insurance Portability and Accountability Act) Privacy Rule that restricts mental institutions and mental healthcare professionals from revealing any information about psychiatric patients. Under HIPAA, their hands are tied from warning the public about the potential dangers posed by patients after their release.

When the Virginia Tech gunman was asked on his application to buy a firearm if he ever had been institutionalized, he lied, and there was no way for the gun seller to check his background for a history of mental health problems which would have prevented him from purchasing the gun that caused so much human misery.

If the histories of such patients were placed in a national data base accessible to those on a need-to-know basis like gun dealers and law enforcement agencies, deranged future criminals would be prevented from arming themselves. But this is only a partial solution. Perpetrators with a history of mental illness or any criminal record for that matter can pay a friend with no record to buy guns for them.

The debate over banning or allowing firearms continues and without a national referendum or a third party to break government gridlock it will never end.

CONCLUSION
Immodest Proposals

Anyone who reads the newspapers or watches the news on TV, even the Fox Channel, must have realized that America is in crisis—or to use the first President Bush's phrase—we are in "deep do-do." The situation has reached critical mass but not nuclear implosion—although we are soon approaching the political equivalent of Chernobyl. Inactive and unresponsive to its constituents for decades, the American government is about to go nuclear—or as the second President Bush's pronounces it, "*nucular.*" (It's worrisome that the man who has his finger on the nuclear button doesn't know how to pronounce it).

This is what's going on … and down:

Two major political parties polarized and paralyzed by partisan faction and an unjustified fear of Evangelical wrath, a clueless President who somehow manages to sleep soundly at night despite the blood of 3,000-plus Americans—and growing—on his hands, corrupt politicians whose interests are more corporate than constituent, a Supreme Court nibbling away at the Bill of Rights and on the verge of resurrecting the nightmare of back-alley abortions, the Christian right obsessed with what goes on in our bedrooms, abortion clinics and bridal chapels, lobbyists and special interests whose power and influence exceeds that of American voters, an unwinnable war that has made the U.S. more, not less, liable to domestic terrorist attacks, political campaigns that sling more dirt than mud wrestling contests, a Third World-level of health insurance coverage that leaves 50 million uninsured Americans literally in peril of their lives, an educational system that hands out high school diplomas to students 20 percent of whom can't read their graduation certificate, crime that is enflamed by the NRA's arming of convicted felons and murderous schizophrenics—all crises this work has offered some help and recommendations for averting before Three Mile Island metastasizes from a spot on the map to a metaphor for our national *malaise*—to use the term that among other disastrous decisions cost Jimmy Carter a second shot at the presidency.

Some of these solutions—such as a national referendum to do the work the legislative and executive branches seem incapable of doing and the founding of a third political party to overcome A) Congressional gridlock, B) an obstructive, veto-rampaging president, and C) Will-Rogers lobbyists who never met a corruptible member of the legislature they didn't like—may seem like pie-in-the-sky panaceas. But remember, in 1854, another embryonic third party—the Republican—had only a handful of members consisting of disaffected Whigs and frustrated abolitionist Democrats. And yet within six years the new party would elect its first President and change the nation's history for the better. (Germany's National Socialist rolls began with only 23 goose-stepping members.)

Providing affordable health insurance for all Americans will cost a modest increase in the current Medicare tax withholding rate from 1.45 percent to 7 to 10 percent—half the 13 to 15 percent rate which the average middle-class employee now pays for private insurance. The new Medicare tax will be unobjectionable to all but the most Paleolithic read-my-lips-no-new-taxes zealots.

The Country You Save May Be Your Own

Hopefully, as this work has already demonstrated, the crises facing the American people are neither intractable nor inevitable.

But the key to their solution rests with you, the average voter, not a do-nothing legislature immobilized by special interest money or a clueless president with what blogger Rick Moran has called a "Messiah complex" who only heeds the counsel of God, Billy Graham and Karl Rove. Bush has said, "I'm the decider," and he's apparently decided that the deaths of 2,000 to 4,000 more Americans in Iraq are justified to prove that his wrong-headed policies toward that devastated nation are right.

What can Mr. Joe or Ms. Jane Citizen do? No radical or impractical time-consuming action is required. You don't have to join the ranks of sociopaths masquerading as anarchists who infiltrate peaceful political marches and throw rocks at SWAT teams, which results in the inevitable police riot.

This work has already suggested myriad solutions, but for those readers with a short attention span, here's a recap:

An end-run around Congressional and executive branch gridlock can be accomplished by the establishment of a third party. Email CNN's maverick political commentator Lou Dobbs at [http://www.cnn.com/CNN/ Programs/lou.dobbs.tonight/^], and ask, no, *beg*, him to publicize the idea of a new party to circumvent the apathy and inertia of our political leaders. Also contact Tim Russert, NBC's brilliant host of *Meet the Press*, for the same purpose at [mtp@msnbc.com.]

Email Nebraska Senator Chuck Hagel at [http://hagel.senate.gov/ index.cfm?FuseAction=Contact.Home], who has already proposed the concept on TV, and urge him to do more than talk to TV reporters about founding a new party.

Email your Congressman or Congresswoman and Senators and threaten to vote them out of office during the next election if they don't get off their Armani-clad butts and bring our imperiled troops home from Iraq and Afghanistan NOW! [To find your Senators' email addresses, contact: http://www.familytreemagazine.com/sen_email.asp. To find your U.S. Representative's email address, contact: http://www.weblsing-erz.com/jhoffman/congress-email.html.]

Don't be afraid to guilt-trip your representatives on Capitol Hill. Remind them that whenever they vote for a war funding bill that fails to tie financing to troop withdrawal, three or more American soldiers die needlessly in Iraq every day. Remind them that the blood of these unfortunate military personnel who only joined the armed forces for college money is on their palms, greased by lobbyists and their corporate paymasters.

You probably won't get a response—or at best, a form letter (which I have received) saying something like, "Thank you for your interest in this [unspecified, natch] issue. Be assured, Congressman X is doing everything possible ..."

No, he's not, or the bloodbath in Iraq, a ballooning deficit that will be our grandchildren's curse, obscene tax cuts for *nouveau grosse* CEOs who blow $6,000 on shower curtains paid for with company money, the continued existence of handguns which end 37,000 American lives per year and which a preponderance of voters say they want taken off the market, crumbling schools infested with guns, drugs and illiterates who hold high school diplomas, a scandalous healthcare situation that leaves 50 million citizens uninsured, a Supreme Court and Evangelicals who want to return women to coat-hanger abortions—and all the other plagues besetting the nation—would at least begin to approach a solution.

If your missives are ignored by your elected representatives, make good on your threat. But you have to find someone to vote for, not just someone to vote against. In most states, when the next election approaches, sample ballots are sent in advance of election day to every registered voter. These brochures not only contain a list of candidates and ballot propositions, but often include a one-page statement by each candidate describing his political platform. Do your homework and read these statements, then vote for the candidate whose political philosophy most nearly reflects your own.

To paraphrase Lenin, "Couch potatoes of the world, unite! You have nothing to lose but your TV remotes." So get off the sofa, stop window-shopping on eBay, put down *The Da Vinci Code*, and start harassing your Congressman and Senators with emails, letters and phone calls.

You may end up *Saving America* in the process.

—Frank Sanello
June 11, 2007

ABOUT THE AUTHORS ...

Adel Nemr Shenouda, M.D., F.A.C.P., is Associate Professor *emeritus* of Nephrology at the University of Tennessee Medical School in Chattanooga. Born in Assiout, Egypt, in 1941, Dr. Shenouda received his medical degree from Cairo University's Medical College where he graduated with honors in 1963. He did his internship at Cairo University Hospital and his residency in internal medicine at the Coptic Hospital in Cairo.

Dr. Shenouda moved to England in 1969 where he completed his residency in internal medicine at Dorking and Redhill Hospitals in Surrey and Peppard Hospital in Oxonshire. From 1971 to 1973, he was Resident in Internal Medicine at the Erlanger Hospital Medical Center in Chattanooga, Tennessee. From 1973 to 1975, he was a Fellow in Nephrology at the University of Tennessee Medical School in Memphis. In 1975, Dr. Shenouda began private practice in Chattanooga and was named Assistant Director of Erlanger's Nephrology Department and the same year Co-Director of the Dialysis Clinic, Inc.

Memorial Hospital appointed him Director of its Acute Dialysis Unit in 1976. The University of Tennessee Medical School named Dr. Shenouda Assistant Professor of Nephrology and Internal Medicine in 1975 and promoted him to Clinical Associate Professor in 1981. The doctor was inducted as a Fellow of the American College of Physicians in 1979. He became Managing Partner For Nephrology Associates and CEO of the Chattanooga Kidney Center in 2001.

As a much respected and beloved member of the medical and local communities, Dr. Shenouda's retirement announcement in 2006 after 32 years of practice made the front page of the Chattanooga Free Press.

A Coptic Orthodox Christian, the future physician attended public schools in his native Egypt, which exposed him to Muslim culture and which he feels gave him a unique insider/outsider perspective on Islam, its customs, theology and politics. As a resident of the United States for the past 36 years, he represents a knowledgeable bridge between East and West.

The father of four and grandfather of two, Dr. Shenouda and his wife Brenda maintain a *pied-à-terre* in Atlanta for weekend getaways and make their home in Chattanooga. Although retired from medical practice, the Professor remains a passionate consumer of current events and a perceptive observer of the American political scene and social issues.

The author can be contacted at <u>ANSHENOUDA@yahoo.com</u>.

*   *   *   *

Nationally known author and syndicated columnist Frank Sanello has written 21 books, including *The Opium Wars: The Addiction of One Empire and the Corruption of Another*, which after its American release was recently published in China; *The Knights Templars: God's Warriors, the Devil's Bankers;* and *To Kill a King: A History of Royal Murders and Assassinations from Ancient Egypt to the Present.* His latest book is *Tweakers: How Crystal Meth Is Ravaging Gay America.*

Sanello is currently writing *Faith and Finance in the Renaissance: The Rise and Ruin of the Fugger Empire*, a centuries-spanning epic about the influential family of bankers and patrons of the arts who were the German equivalent of their contemporaries, the Medici.

Upcoming books include *Soap: A History of How the World Cleaned Up Its Act* and *Hitler's Vicar: The Roman Catholic Priest Who Ruled Slovakia for Nazi Germany.*

A journalist for the past 26 years, Sanello has written articles for the *Washington Post*, the *Los Angeles Times*, the *Chicago Tribune*, the *Boston*

Globe, the *New York Times Syndicate, USA Today, Redbook, People, US Weekly, Penthouse and Cosmo.*

Sanello was formerly a film critic for the *Los Angeles Daily News* and a business reporter for UPI.

The author graduated *cum laude* from the University of Chicago and earned a master's degree from UCLA's film school. He also holds a purple belt in Tae Kwon Do and has volunteered as a kickboxing instructor at AIDS Project Los Angeles where he teaches self-defense to HIV/AIDS patients.

Sanello lives in West Hollywood, California, and can be contacted at FSanello@aol.com.

978-0-595-48013-5
0-595-48013-6

www.ingramcontent.com/pod-product-compliance
Lightning Source LLC
Chambersburg PA
CBHW020423290526
45785CB00002B/702